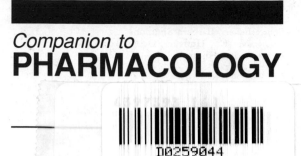

Companion to
PHARMACOLOGY

'000

For Churchill Livingstone:

Publisher Laurence Hunter
Project Editor Barbara Simmons
Production Kay Hunston, Debra Barrie
Designer Ian Hunter

Companion to
PHARMACOLOGY

A Study Guide for self-assessment and revision

M.M. Dale MB BCh PhD

Senior Teaching Fellow
Department of Pharmacology
University of Oxford;
Honorary Lecturer
Department of Pharmacology
University College
London

A.H. Dickenson BSc PhD

Professor of Neuropharmacology
Department of Pharmacology
University College
London

D.G. Haylett BSc PhD

Senior Lecturer
Department of Pharmacology
University College
London

SECOND EDITION

CHURCHILL LIVINGSTONE
NEW YORK EDINBURGH LONDON MADRID MELBOURNE SAN FRANCISCO AND TOKYO 1995

CHURCHILL LIVINGSTONE
Medical Division of Pearson Professional Limited

Distributed in the United States of America by Churchill
Livingstone Inc., 650 Avenue of the Americas, New
York, N.Y. 10011, and by associated companies,
branches and representatives throughout the world.

First edition 1993
Second edition 1995

ISBN 0 443 053855

British Library Cataloguing in Publication Data
A catalogue record for this book is available from the
British Library.

Library of Congress Cataloging in Publication Data
A catalog record for this book is available from the
Library of Congress.

Whilst the advice and information in this book is
believed to be true and accurate at the date of going to
press, neither the authors nor the publisher can accept
any legal responsibility or liability for any errors or
omissions that may be made. In particular (but without
limiting the generality of the preceding disclaimer) every
effort has been made to check indications for drug use
and any drug dosages; however it is still possible that
errors have been missed. In addition indications for drug
use and dosage schedules are being constantly revised
and new side effects recognised. The reader is thus
strongly urged to directly consult the drug companies'
printed instructions before administering any of the
drugs suggested in this book.

The right of Dr M.M. Dale, Professor A.H. Dickenson
and Dr D.G. Haylett to be identified as the authors of
this Work has been asserted by them in accordance with
the Copyright, Designs and Patents Act 1988.

The
publisher's
policy is to use
**paper manufactured
from sustainable forests**

Typesetting by IMH (Cartrif), Loanhead, Scotland
Printed in Singapore

Preface

Pharmacology is not a conceptually difficult science — it does not have the barriers of abstruse thought that characterise, for example, theoretical physics or higher mathematics. The problem in learning pharmacology is that there are a great many disparate facts and ideas which have to be mastered, along with a multitude of complex and hard-to-remember drug names. The subject is usually taught in terms of systems (e.g. the pharmacology of the central nervous system, the cardiovascular system, the gastro-intestinal system), the information being neatly compartmentalised. But when it is necessary to use this information at the bedside or in the experimental laboratory, it is rarely sufficient, and in fact it may be a hindrance to think only in terms of these tidy compartments. Thus a clinical student attending a patient who had developed deep vein thrombosis and pulmonary embolism after an abdominal operation, may have to consider not only the anticoagulant therapy, sedation and analgesia required, but also the effects of the drugs which will have been given for premedication, the anaesthetics and neuromuscular-blocking agents used during the operation, the antibiotics which may have been administered, as well as any agents which might have been employed to clear the bowels before the operation and to treat the paralytic ileus or decreased bladder function afterwards. Similarly, a pharmacology postgraduate, working with in vitro preparations of lung as part of an asthma research project, may need to bear in mind the pharmacological responses not only of bronchiolar smooth muscle but also of vascular tissue, endothelium, mast cells, leucocytes, sympathetic neurons, autonomic ganglia, parasympathetic neurons or peptide co-transmitters.

One of the main problems of learning pharmacology is thus that, in addition to understanding the subject matter, it is necessary to become sufficiently familiar with it so that one can, as it were, manoeuvre amongst the facts and ideas of the subject and readily appreciate and recall relevant interrelationships. An efficient way of accomplishing this is to work through the material several times, meeting and considering the facts and concepts in different contexts. The aim of this book is to assist in this process. It is based on *Pharmacology* by Rang, Dale and Ritter and would be most effectively used in conjunction with this textbook, but could be used on its own or in conjunction with another book.

The text is divided into two parts. Part 1 contains 44 minichapters, 43 of these corresponding to the 43 chapters of *Pharmacology*. In each of these, some background material is given, then a series of questions on the subject matter covered in the relevant chapter in the main book, followed by the answers. Chapter 44 is on smooth muscle and in it we pull together information on the action of mediators/transmitters/drugs from several areas of pharmacology, relating their action to modern concepts of the mechanisms for contraction and relaxation. (This chapter is likely to be of interest mainly to pharmacology students.) Part 2 has two sections. The first consists of questions and, to answer these, it is necessary to collate ideas and information from several chapters of *Pharmacology* or from other sources. The second section of Part 2 contains the answers to these general questions, several of them in chart or diagram form.

In dealing with some topics, we have emphasised signal-transduction mechanisms. We feel that knowledge in this area is progressing so rapidly that it is now important that the subject matter of pharmacology includes not just a consideration of the stimulus (drug/transmitter/mediator) and response, but also the stimulus–response coupling mechanisms.

Further, in order to help with the problem of the dauntingly large number of drug names faced by the students learning pharmacology, we have included, as an appendix, a list of important drugs, divided into agents of primary and secondary importance. The list is based on one issued at University College London some years ago, updated with reference not only to *Pharmacology* but to the British National Formulary.

We should emphasise that it is not expected that students will memorise the answers to the questions in either Part 1 or Part 2; however, the process of thinking about them should help students to acquire facility in finding their way among the facts and ideas of pharmacology. The answers to the very general questions in Part 2 should enable the reader to correlate — often in clinical context — information learned in separate, tidy compartments, while the summary charts and diagrams used throughout this book should be useful in revision.

The main object of this Companion, then, is to assist students to work through the subject matter of pharmacology on their own and achieve an integrated understanding of it, but it might also be of value in preparing for examinations, which is, after all, not an unacceptable aim.

London
1995

M.M. Dale
A.H. Dickenson
D.G. Haylett

Acknowledgements

While emphasising that any errors in this book are our own, we wish to acknowledge the useful advice and constructive criticism of our colleagues: Dr C. Twort, Dr R.A. Webster, Professor D.H. Jenkinson, Dr R.E. Muid, Dr J.C. Foreman, Professor H.P. Rang, Professor D. Colquhoun, Professor S.G. Cull-Candy, Dr C. Stanford, Professor J.M. Ritter, Professor J. Mandelstam, and students Peter Hill and Louise Stanfa.

List of figures

Contents

NOTE:

All references to pages, tables or illustrations in *Pharmacology* 3rd edn (Rang, Dale and Ritter, Churchill Livingstone, 1995) are denoted by the symbol 📖.

Otherwise page references refer to other sections of this book.

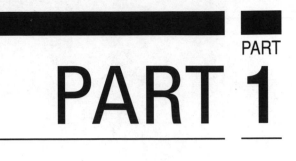

PART

PART 1

1

How drugs act: general principles

BACKGROUND INFORMATION

Most drugs act by binding to target molecules which may be enzymes, carriers, ion channels or receptors. In most cases the combination is reversible, and the drug–receptor complex dissociates readily. Specificity of action depends on the fact that individual classes of drugs bind only to particular targets and the targets in turn recognise only those classes of drug. The four types of target are distinct and separate; thus for example, in pharmacological parlance, an enzyme is not regarded as a receptor. The concept of classifying drugs in terms of their action on receptors is central in pharmacology.

The binding of drug to receptor obeys the Law of Mass Action. At equilibrium, drug *occupancy* of a receptor is related to the *drug concentration* by the Hill–Langmuir equation. The greater the *affinity* of drug for receptor, the lower the concentration range over which it will approach saturation of the receptors.

A drug which acts on a receptor to produce a response is termed an agonist; such a drug may be a full agonist or a partial agonist. A drug which prevents the action of an agonist on a receptor is termed an antagonist.

In a more general sense *antagonism* between two drugs can occur by various mechanisms:

- competitive antagonism at the receptor
- block of receptor–effector linkage (non-competitive antagonism)
- pharmacokinetic antagonism
- physiological antagonism
- chemical antagonism.

An agonist's potency depends on both its *affinity* for the receptor and its efficacy.

QUESTIONS

1. **a.** Explain what is meant by the term 'receptor'.

   b. Can an enzyme be regarded as a receptor? If not, explain why.

2. What is meant by 'efficacy'?

3. What is meant by 'affinity'?

4. What is meant by 'spare receptors'?

5. What is the efficacy of the competitive antagonist **atropine** for muscarinic receptors?

6. **a.** What simple model represents the reaction of drug with receptor?

   b. On the basis of the model, and applying the Law of Mass Action, define the equilibrium constant, K_A.

   c. What equation relates the proportion of receptors occupied, p_A, to the drug concentration and the equilibrium constant, K_A?

7. What is the relationship between the *affinity* of a drug for a receptor, and the *equilibrium constant, K_A*, for the interaction of that drug with the receptor?

8. The magnitude of the response to a drug (e.g. the response of guinea-pig ileum

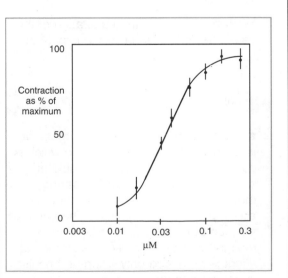

Fig. 1 The concentration–response curve of the effect of histamine on guinea-pig ileum.

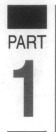

PART

1

smooth muscle to histamine) is related to the number of receptors occupied. Figure 1 depicts an experimentally observed concentration–response curve (note the logarithmic concentration scale). Could such a graph be used to give a measure of the affinity of **histamine** for the histamine receptors on guinea-pig ileum smooth muscle?

9. What is the difference between 'reversible' and 'irreversible' competitive antagonism?

10. What is meant by the term 'dose-ratio'? How is it related to concentration of the antagonist?

11. How might the affinity of a reversible competitive antagonist for a receptor be measured? What is the general significance of the fact that the affinity of reversible competitive antagonists can be accurately measured?

12. What is the difference between a full agonist and a partial agonist? Draw a rough graph showing how the relationship between occupancy and response might differ for a full and a partial agonist, expressing the response as a percentage of maximum on the ordinate and the proportion of receptors occupied (on a scale of 0–1) on the abscissa.

13. What processes, due to alteration of the receptors, might underlie the loss of the response to a drug?

ANSWERS

1. **a.** In pharmacology, the term, receptor, is defined as a protein molecule which is part of a cell and which is capable of selectively binding a drug, hormone, mediator, or neurotransmitter, thereby eliciting a cellular response. The principal function of a receptor is to serve as a recognition site. With most receptors, an effect is produced only when an agonist is bound, otherwise the receptor is functionally inactive; however, some

receptors, e.g. benzodiazepine receptors, are exceptions to this general rule (see below). Drugs which are *agonists* activate receptors; drugs which are *antagonists* interact with receptors without activating them, but in so doing prevent activation by agonists. *Activation* of a receptor involves setting in train the series of events which leads to the response of the cell by: (i) the opening of an integral ion channel; (ii) the initiation of enzyme activity, either directly or through G-protein coupling; or (iii) interaction of the ligand–receptor complex with DNA and subsequent modification of transcription. (Note that some receptors, e.g. benzodiazepine receptors, have a resting activity— agonists increase and inverse agonists decrease this activity; both effects can be blocked by antagonists.) [See 📄 p. 635.]

b. In pharmacological parlance, *an enzyme is not regarded as a receptor*. An enzyme is a protein catalyst of a biochemical reaction. It need not be part of a cell (though it frequently is) and it need not initiate a cellular response. An enzyme also recognises and binds specifically with a chemical substance, in this case a substrate; *but in the process, the substrate is altered, giving rise to reaction products*. This does not occur with a receptor, as defined in pharmacology. Analysis of the relationship between the concentration of substrate and the velocity of an *enzyme reaction* involves using the Michaelis– Menten equation. In the case of *enzyme reactions*, both competitive inhibition by substrate competition and non-competitive inhibition are evaluated by Lineweaver–Burk plots. Lineweaver–Burk plots are not appropriate for the analysis of drug–**receptor** interactions; most pharmacologists use Schild plots for the evaluation of competitive antagonism at a receptor. (The advantage of a Schild plot is that it uses a null method—equal occupancies in both the presence and absence of competitive antagonists are assumed to produce equal responses.) [See Answer 11 below and 🗎 p. 8.]

(Some confusion regarding the difference between receptors and enzymes may arise from the fact that some membrane receptors (e.g. tyrosine–kinase-linked receptors) may have enzyme activity, in that they have an integral catalytic domain. However, the catalytic domain in these receptors is quite separate from the domain which recognises and binds the ligand. The intracellular enzymic domain of the receptor does not interact with the ligand at all, but catalyses quite separate reactions within the cell, namely phosphorylation of tyrosine residues (which may be on the intracellular portion of the receptor itself).

2. The ability of a drug when bound to a receptor to initiate a cell response [see 🗎 p. 13 box].

3. The affinity of a drug for a receptor is, put simply, the tendency of that drug to bind to that receptor. (The affinity constant has the dimensions of concentration^{-1}.) [See Answer 6 below and 🗎 p. 9 box.]

4. The existence of more receptors in a tissue than are required to be occupied by an agonist for a full response [see 🗎 p. 13].

5. Zero. The efficacy of *all* competitive antagonists is zero, since efficacy is the ability of a drug to initiate a response when bound to a receptor, and a competitive antagonist such as **atropine**, by definition, does not itself initiate a response [see 🗎 p. 13 box].

6. **a.** The model would be:

$$A + R \underset{k_{-1}}{\overset{k_{+1}}{\rightleftharpoons}} AR$$

Where A is the drug, R represents free receptors, and AR is the drug–receptor complex.

b. $K_A = \dfrac{k_{-1}}{k_{+1}}$

and at equilibrium, $K_A = \dfrac{[A][R]}{[AR]}$

c. $p_A = \dfrac{[A]}{K_A + [A]}$

[see 🗎 pp. 7–9].

7. The affinity of a drug for a receptor is inversely related to the equilibrium constant K_A, i.e. the higher the affinity of the drug for the receptors, the lower the K_A [see 🗎 p. 8].

8. No. Although *occupancy* by agonist is related to concentration, by the Hill–Langmuir equation, the relation between agonist occupancy and response is usually unknown and expected to be complex and non-linear.

9. In competitive antagonism there is competition between agonist and antagonist for the receptor. The antagonism may be *reversible* or *irreversible*. With reversible antagonism, the block by the antagonist can be surmounted by increasing the concentration of the agonist. In this case, in the presence of the antagonist, the agonist log-concentration–response curve is shifted to the right with no change in slope or maximum [see Fig. 2 and 🗎 Figs 1.3, 1.10]. With an irreversible competitive antagonist, increasing the concentration of the antagonist has a very different effect on the concentration–effect curve of the agonist [see 🗎 Fig. 1.10]. It is important to know and understand the definition of competitive antagonism.

10. The term, dose-ratio, refers to the shift of the concentration–effect curve of an agonist in the presence of a reversible competitive antagonist [see Answer 8 above and 🗎 p. 10 box]. Thus in Figure 2 for concentration of antagonist, B1, the dose-ratio (r) is A1/A0, for concentration of antagonist, B2, it is A2/A0, and so on. The dose-ratio increases in linear fashion with increasing concentration of reversible competitive antagonist [see 🗎 p. 10, Fig. 1.3B].

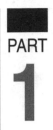

PART

1

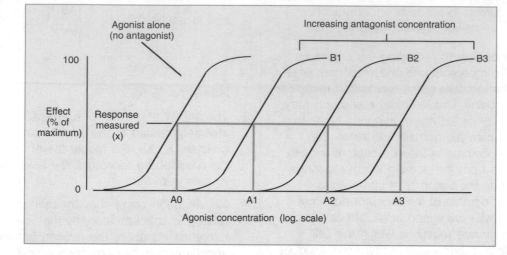

Fig. 2 Schematic graph of the log of agonist concentration versus response (% of maximum), showing the effect of increasing concentrations (B1, B2, B3) of a reversible competitive antagonist on the concentration–response curve of the agonist, namely parallel displacement of the curve with no decrease in maximum. The extent of the shift can be expressed as a dose-ratio [defined as the factor by which the agonist concentration must be increased to restore a given response (x above)]. Thus for antagonist concentration B1, the dose-ratio r = A1/A0; for antagonist concentration B2, r = A2/A0 and so on. The dose-ratio increases linearly with antagonist concentration.

11. The equilibrium dissociation constant, K_B, for the receptor–antagonist interaction can be obtained from the relation between the dose-ratio (r) and the antagonist concentration, which is expressed as:

$$r - 1 = \frac{[B]}{K_B}$$

This is the Schild equation. K_B can be derived from a Schild plot, the graphical representation of the Schild equation [see 📖 p. 10, Fig. 1.3].

Equilibrium dissociation constants can also be obtained from radioligand-binding studies [see 📖 p. 13].

The measurement of the affinity of reversible competitive antagonists has been extensively used to classify receptors. For example, the differences in the affinity of **mepyramine** in different tissues led Ash and Schild to suggest that there were different types of histamine receptors in the tissues concerned.

12. See Figure 3, which shows the relationship between occupancy and response for a full agonist and a partial agonist (as well as for an antagonist) based on the theoretical curves in 📖 Figure 1.5A. Note that in Figure 3 the 'transducer function' is assumed to be hyperbolic. The key points are:

1. that, even with 100% occupancy, the partial agonist fails to produce a maximum response, and

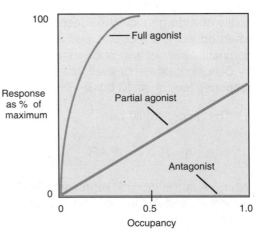

Fig. 3 Schematic figure of the relationship between response and occupancy for a full agonist, a partial agonist and an antagonist.

2. that the full agonist may produce a maximum response with only a small proportion of receptors occupied.

[This subject is dealt with in more detail in 🖉 pp. 12–13.]

13. Briefly, the receptors may be uncoupled from the transduction events and/or they may be lost. This last usually involves endocytosis of the ligand–receptor complex [see 🖉 pp. 19–20].

2

How drugs act: molecular aspects

BACKGROUND INFORMATION

Drugs and mediators produce their action in the body by acting on: receptors, ion channels, carrier molecules or enzymes.

Receptors are of four types:

- Situated in the membrane and directly coupled to an ion channel. These receptors cause extremely rapid cell activation with a timescale of milliseconds, e.g. the **acetylcholine** nicotinic receptor.
- Situated in the membrane and coupled via a G-protein to an enzyme or ion channel, e.g. **adrenaline** on β_2-receptors in smooth muscle activates adenylate cyclase, **noradrenaline** on α_1-receptors in smooth muscle activates phospholipase C, **bradykinin** in fibroblasts activates phospholipase A_2—all being coupled to their respective enzymes by G-proteins. Cardiac muscarinic receptors are coupled by G-proteins to potassium channels. These receptors cause rather slower cell activation, with a timescale of seconds.
- Situated in the membrane and having either integral tyrosine kinase activity (e.g. the **insulin** receptor and receptors for various **growth factors**) or becoming linked to tyrosine kinase when a ligand binds (e.g. some **cytokine** receptors). Dimerisation and incestuous phosphorylation occur. These receptors usually cause even slower cell activation with a timescale of minutes, e.g. the insulin receptor, but some are involved in more rapid responses, e.g. the **fMetLeuPhe** receptor on neutrophils.
- Situated in the cytosol or nucleus, with the ligand–receptor complex acting on DNA resulting in (i) transcription and translation of mediator proteins, or (ii) repression of

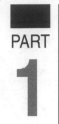

expression of certain genes with inhibition of production of specific proteins. These receptors cause cell activation with a timescale of minutes to hours, e.g. the glucocorticoid, **hydrocortisone**.

Many receptor proteins have now been isolated and characterised and the genes have been cloned.

Ion channels can be affected by drugs such as **local anaesthetics** which physically block the sodium channel, or by agents such as the **calcium channel antagonists**, which bind to specific sites in the calcium channel protein, inhibiting channel opening, or by agents such as the **benzodiazepines** which bind elsewhere on the receptor–channel complex of the chloride channel facilitating its opening by the neurotransmitter GABA.

Carrier molecules, which transport ions and small organic molecules into or out of cells, can be affected by drugs which inhibit them, e.g. **loop diuretics** on the $Na^+/K^+/2Cl^-$ co-transporter in the loop of Henle.

Drug action on enzymes is usually inhibitory, e.g. **neostigmine** on acetylcholinesterase (an extracellular enzyme) or **iproniazid** on monoamine oxidase (an intracellular enzyme). The action is usually direct, often by substrate competition but sometimes by inactivation, e.g. **aspirin** on cyclo-oxygenase. Some drugs inhibit enzymes indirectly, e.g. **heparin** inhibits the coagulation enzymes by speeding up the action of a natural inhibitor, antithrombin III. Some drugs can themselves develop enzyme activity, e.g. **anistreplase**.

G-proteins

G-proteins consist of three subunits: α (which in the resting state has GDP bound to it), β and γ. The β and γ subunits anchor the protein in the membrane. When a ligand interacts with a receptor there is a conformational change in the receptor such that it acquires affinity for the G-protein, which binds. The GDP associated with the α subunit is exchanged for GTP, which activates the G-protein. The α subunit now dissociates from the receptor and can interact with a target (an enzyme or ion channel) causing activation or inactivation. The effect is terminated when the bound GTP is hydrolysed,

allowing the α subunit to recombine with $\beta\gamma$. Specificity of receptor function may be dependent on specificity of the α subunits. A transducer function of the $\beta\gamma$ subunits is being increasingly recognised. The activity of some enzymes (e.g. adenylate cyclase) can be modulated by both inhibitory and stimulatory G-proteins.

Intracellular messenger systems

The main intracellular messenger systems are:

- The adenylate cyclase system, which increases cAMP generation. The cAMP activates various cAMP-dependent protein kinases (PKAs) which phosphorylate various intracellular proteins (e.g. enzymes) regulating their function by activating or inactivating them.
- The guanylyl cyclase system which increases cGMP generation. The cGMP activates a protein kinase (PKG) which, like PKA, phosphorylates various proteins regulating their function.
- The phospholipase C (PLC) and phospholipase D (PLD) systems. PLC acts on phosphatidylinositol bisphosphate (PIP_2) to give $InsP_3$, which mobilises intracellular calcium, and DAG, which activates protein kinase C (PKC). The increased calcium initiates various events in different cell types (e.g. contraction in smooth muscle, secretion in glands). It may combine with calmodulin to activate enzymes. PKC, like PKA, regulates the function of a variety of proteins by phosphorylating them. The $InsP_3$ and DAG derived from PIP_2 by PLC action usually have only transient existence. DAG can also be generated, less transiently, by phospholipase D (PLD) action on phosphatidylcholine (PC) to give phosphatidic acid (PA) which can be converted to DAG [see p. 41, Fig. 2.15].
- The phospholipase A_2 (PLA_2) system. This generates arachidonate (from which the eicosanoids are formed) and is involved in the production of platelet activating factor (PAF). Compounds generated by PLA_2 are important extracellular mediators [see p. 230, Fig. 11.5] but some (e.g. arachidonate itself) may function as intracellular messengers in some cells.

QUESTIONS

Most questions on the molecular aspects of drug action are in Part 2 and are best attempted when the reader is more conversant with drug action in general.

1. What is the evidence that the receptor for **acetylcholine** at the neuromuscular junction is part of the ion channel and that the acetylcholine-mediated increase in sodium and potassium permeability is thus caused directly and not by second messenger generation?

2. **a.** What is the evidence that agonists can increase intracellular calcium ion concentration?

   b. What is the mechanism of this action?

3. Indicate which of the following statements are true and which are false. If you think a statement is false, explain why.

   A. Cholera toxin has proved to be a useful tool in analysing G-protein function since it acts only on inhibitory G-proteins (G_i), causing persistent activation.

   B. Membrane receptors are proteins embedded in the plasma membrane having extracellular domains which bind ligands, but no intracellular domains.

   C. Most G-protein-coupled receptors (though including the receptors for a wide variety of transmitters, mediators and drugs) are similar in structure, comprising seven membrane-spanning domains.

   D. Receptors can activate enzymes through G-proteins but by definition do not themselves have any enzyme activity.

ANSWERS

1. The response is far too fast for second messengers to be involved, reaching a peak in a fraction of a millisecond [see 📖 p. 31].

2. **a.** The rise in $[Ca^{2+}]_i$ can be measured by fluorescence indicators such as Fura-2 [see 📖 p. 39.]

   b. $InsP_3$ acts on a calcium channel on the membrane of the sarcoplasmic reticulum to release stored Ca^{2+} in a series of bursts. There may also be receptor-operated Ca^{2+} channels in the plasma membrane [see 📖 p. 39].

3. **A.** False; it acts on G_s, causing persistent activation. Pertussis toxin acts on G_i [see 📖 p. 35].

   B. False on two counts; all have intracellular domains and the ligand-binding domains of G-protein-coupled receptors are within the membrane, not extracellular [see 📖 Fig. 2.4B].

   C. True [see 📖 p. 29, Fig. 2.4B].

   D. False; in tyrosine-kinase-linked receptors, the tyrosine kinase is part of the receptor structure though separate from the ligand-binding domain [see 📖 p. 43 box, Fig. 2.4C].

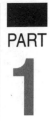

PART

1

3

Measurement in pharmacology

BACKGROUND INFORMATION

It is essential to be able to measure accurately the effects of drugs, either to compare quantitatively the effects of different substances or to study the action of a single substance under different circumstances. It is also important to be able to identify and measure the concentration of mediators/drugs/hormones in body fluids or of pharmacologically active agents in extracts of plants, bacterial cultures, snake venoms, etc. Bioassays are used for these purposes. Increasingly, it is becoming possible to measure drugs/mediators/transmitters, etc., by chemical techniques. These methods are inherently more accurate and, where possible, are supplanting bioassays.

QUESTIONS

1. Define the term 'bioassay'.

2. Give five uses of a bioassay.

3. What is the difference between a 'quantal' and a 'graded' response?

4. Give examples of drugs for which bioassays are necessary to measure activity or for the biological standardisation.

5. What is the difference between a direct and an indirect assay?

6. What should be inherent in the design of a bioassay?

7. What is meant by 95% confidence limits?

8. In some straightforward direct assays (such as that described in the answer to 5 above) one obtains the individually effective dose for each animal. In some

assays involving all-or-none responses, this is not possible.

For example, in assaying a new painkilling drug in rats, one procedure for testing analgesia is to hold a rat gently so that its tail is draped across a slit in a board with a source of heat on the other side. After 15 seconds, the sensation of warmth begins to feel painful. The end point of the assay is the flick of the tail away from the slit. Analgesia is considered to be present if the tail is not flicked away within 15 seconds, an all-or-none response. But unlike the assay with digitalis on frogs, one cannot infuse the analgesic into the rats under test until the end point is reached. What procedures can be adopted to measure the potency of a new analgesic in this situation?

9. In a clinical trial what are the important factors which must be considered to avoid bias?

10. What is a placebo?

11. Apart from the ethical problems, what are the three main faults with LD_{50} measurements?

12. Other than on the football field, what is a yellow card used for?

13. **a.** What is the Therapeutic Index?

    b. Why is it not a very useful measure of clinical safety?

14. Name the three main types of chemical assays of drugs/mediators/transmitters.

ANSWERS

1. Bioassay is the ozone-friendly measurement of the concentration or potency of an unknown drug by measuring the biological response it produces. Comparison with a 'standard' drug is necessary [see 📖 p. 52 box].

2. **a.** To measure the pharmacological activity of new agents.

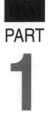

b. To measure the concentration of known substances, e.g. the concentration of heparin in an extract of hog stomach.

c. To study the function of endogenous chemical mediators.

d. To measure the clinical effectiveness of a treatment.

e. To measure the toxicity of a drug.

[See 🖊 p. 47.]

3. A quantal response is an all-or-none response, e.g. cessation of the heart beat, a twitch in response to a painful stimulus. This contrasts with a response which is graded and can vary, such as the contraction of a strip of guinea-pig ileum, a change in blood pressure, or the length of time it takes an individual to answer a series of mathematical questions [see 🖊 p. 52].

4. Some examples are **insulin**, **corticotrophin**, **digitalis** and **heparin**.

5. A *direct* assay can be performed only if there is a fixed end point (as with a quantal response), in which case the dose or concentration of both the unknown drug and the standard required to reach the end point can be measured *directly* and compared. For example, if a standard preparation of digitalis is infused into each of 50 anaesthetised frogs until the heart stops, and the same procedure is carried out with a preparation of foxglove (concentration of **digitalis** unknown), a measurement of the mean volume of each which is necessary to reach the end point can be obtained. Since one knows the concentration of digitalis in the standard preparation, one can calculate directly the concentration of digitalis in the unknown. Note that one obtains the results in units of drug. (This type of assay, involving the killing of large numbers of frogs, is in fact no longer done. But an assay based on the same principles is used, e.g. to measure and standardise **heparin** preparations.)

Another example of a direct type of assay is the old-fashioned matching assay.

Indirect assays are based on graded responses. Here one does not obtain one's measurement in units of drug and thus obtain a direct estimate of the potency of the unknown. One measures units of *response* and must therefore know the relationship between the two, i.e. one must construct a dose–response curve for both unknown and standard. If the responses of both standard and unknown are plotted against the logarithm of dose, parallel curves should be obtained. The midportion of each dose–response curve is linear and this enables one to read off the potency ratio [see 🖊 p. 50].

6. Minimal biological variation, the avoidance of systematic errors, ability to estimate the errors of the results and comparison of the unknown with a standard [see 🖊 p. 50].

7. The limits into which 95% of the results would be expected to fall if the experiment were repeated many times [see 🖊 p. 50].

8. One procedure would be to use, say, four groups of rats, with 10 in each group, and to inject each group with a different bolus dose of the standard analgesic, usually morphine. One might obtain a result in which two rats manifested analgesia (according to the criteria given in Question 8) at the lowest dose, four with the next higher dose, six with the next higher dose, and nine with the highest dose. One could then construct a log dose–response curve of analgesia with the standard drug. If one carried out similar measurements using the unknown analgesic, one would have generated two dose-response curves and could calculate the relative potency of the unknown drug [see 🖊 Figs 3.2, 3.3A].

9. **a.** Randomisation of the patients with regard to age, sex, severity of the disease, etc.

b. A double blind technique for administering drugs and assessing response of the patients.

c. Appropriate statistical interpretation of the results [see 🖊 p. 57 box].

10. An inert tablet, or injection, used in a clinical trial for comparison with an active drug.

11. **a.** Only death is measured—an extreme end point which avoids sublethal effects.

    b. Species differences are considerable.

    c. Only short-term toxicity is gauged, not the long-term effects of a drug [see 🖊 p. 57].

12. A voluntary reporting by doctors of adverse effects of a drug—usually a drug recently introduced into clinical practice [see 🖊 p. 59].

13. **a.** One commonly used definition is Therapeutic Index = LD_{50}/ED_{50}.

    b. Firstly, because of the problems with LD_{50} (see 11 above), secondly, because the ED_{50} for any drug will vary depending on its clinical use or the severity of the disorder, and finally, because it does not take account of idiosyncratic reactions to drugs.

14. **a.** Radioimmunoassay.

    b. Chromatographic techniques.

    c. Fluorimetric techniques.

    [See 🖊 p. 60.]

4

Absorption, distribution and elimination of drugs

BACKGROUND INFORMATION

The effects of a drug on a patient are dependent not only on the pharmacological effect of the drug but on how the drug is handled in the body. Members of a particular class of drug may have very specific actions on a single receptor population (e.g. the opiate analgesics act on the mu (μ) opioid receptor) but a dose of one specific drug within this class may have no effect, whereas the same dose of another drug acting on the same receptor could cause rapid respiratory depression and death. One reason for this is the ability of the second drug to reach the receptor site, and this is where pharmacokinetics comes in. The main determinants of the fate of a drug are the translocation of the drug molecules in the body and the transformation and subsequent removal of the molecule.

QUESTIONS

Many of the questions on the absorption, distribution and fate of individual drugs are in Part 2 and are best attempted when the reader knows more about drug action.

1. Define 'pharmacokinetics' and 'pharmacodynamics'.

2. **a.** Name four processes by which molecules cross cell membranes.

   b. Which two routes would you pick as being the most important?

3. What properties of a drug determine how well it diffuses across the lipid regions of cell membranes?

4. What is meant by the following terms:

   a. Permeability coefficient?

b. Partition coefficient?

c. Diffusion coefficient?

5. a. Why is the state of ionisation of a drug important?

b. How is the degree of ionisation related to pH?

6. **Morphine** is a weak base (pKa = 8); how would this affect its ionisation in, and absorption from, the stomach (pH about 2) after oral administration?

7. How could you increase excretion of a weak acid?

8. What effect does body fat have on the pharmacokinetics of a highly lipid-soluble drug?

9. a. How does plasma protein binding affect drug distribution and action?

b. Under what circumstances would the displacement of one drug by another be clinically important?

10. What is meant by bioavailability?

11. What is meant by the volume of distribution of a drug?

12. What are the five major compartments important in distribution of a drug?

13. a. What, broadly, are phase I and phase II reactions in drug metabolism?

b. What, in general, are the pharmacokinetic properties and biological properties of phase I and phase II products?

14. What is the P-450 system?

15. What are the consequences of the induction of microsomal enzymes?

16. What is meant by 'first-pass metabolism'?

17. What are the three renal processes which determine how much of a drug is excreted in the urine?

18. a. What factors determine whether there is glomerular filtration of a drug?

b. What determines whether a drug in the filtrate is reabsorbed?

19. What is renal clearance?

20. What is meant by enterohepatic circulation of drugs?

21. What is meant by the plasma steady-state concentration? Is this affected by the doses of drug given?

22. a. What is the plasma half-life ($t_{1/2}$) of a drug?

b. Is it clinically useful to know the plasma half-life of a drug?

23. Why are loading doses of a drug used and under what circumstances?

24. What is meant by 'saturation kinetics' (zero-order kinetics)? Why might it be important to know whether the metabolism of a drug follows saturation kinetics?

25. If drug A, which is being given long term and whose elimination follows first-order kinetics, has reached steady-state plasma concentration, and a second drug, B, which induces the metabolising enzymes for drug A, is then added to the therapeutic regime, will this affect the plasma steady-state concentration of drug A? If so, how? How must the administration of drug A be altered to reach the original steady-state plasma concentration? On a theoretical basis, how long will this take?

ANSWERS

1. Pharmacokinetics is concerned with translocation, chemical transformation and excretion (what the body does to a drug).

   Pharmacodynamics is concerned with the effects of drugs on the body (what drugs do to the body).

2. a. Diffusion through the lipid regions of the cell membrane, diffusion through aqueous pores, carrier-mediated movement and finally pinocytosis [see p. 67].

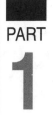

11

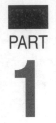

PART

1

b. The first and third are most important since aqueous pores are too small to allow most drugs through, and pinocytosis, although important for macromolecules such as insulin, is not relevant for most drugs [see 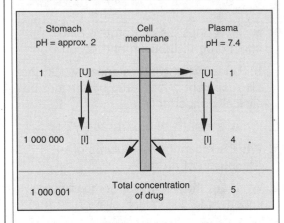 p. 67].

3. Its lipid solubility and the degree of ionisation.

4. **a.** A measure of the number of molecules crossing a membrane per unit of time, area and concentration difference.

   b. A measure of the lipid–aqueous distribution of a drug.

   c. A measure of mobility of molecules in solution (either lipid or aqueous).

   [See p. 68.]

5. **a.** Because only the unionised moiety is lipid-soluble.

   b. The ratio of the ionised (I) and unionised (U) forms varies with pH and can be calculated from the Henderson–Hasselbalch equation.

   For a weak acid $\dfrac{[I]}{[U]} = 10^{\,pH\,-pKa}$

   For a weak base $\dfrac{[I]}{[U]} = 10^{pKa\,-pH}$

   [see pp. 68–69].

6. In the acidic environment of the stomach, most of the **morphine** (pKa = 8) will be ionised and consequently very poorly absorbed [see Fig. 4 and p. 75, Fig. 4.8].

7. Excretion of a weak acid will be increased by making the urine more alkaline. This will result in more of the drug being ionised and therefore lipid-insoluble and thus not available for reabsorption from the renal tubule [see p. 71 box].

8. It can act as a reservoir, since highly lipid-soluble agents will diffuse into fat in large amounts and then be released slowly [see p. 82 box].

For a weak base $\dfrac{[I]}{[U]} = 10^{\,pKa\,-\,pH}$

For morphine (pKa 8) the situation would be as follows:-

in the stomach (pH about 2), the ratio of ionised [I] to unionised [U] drug would be:

$$\frac{[I]}{[U]} = \frac{10^{\,8-2}}{1} = \frac{10^{6}}{1} = \frac{1\,000\,000}{1}$$

in the plasma, (pH 7.4), the ratio would be:

$$\frac{[I]}{[U]} = \frac{10^{\,8-7.4}}{1} = \text{approx.} \ \frac{4}{1}$$

Only a minute proportion of the morphine in the stomach would be in the unionised, lipophilic form, thus absorption from the stomach would be insignificant, and an "ion-trapping" equilibrium may be set up as follows:

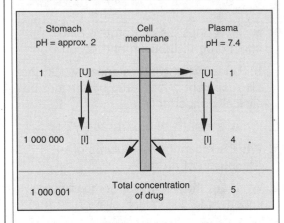

Thus a high proportion of the morphine would be retained in the stomach following oral administration. Even parenterally administered morphine would accumulate in the stomach. Absorption of morphine would occur rather more readily from the intestine where the pH is higher.

Fig. 4 The effect of pH on the absorption of a weak base from the stomach.

9. **a.** Plasma protein binding has several consequences:

   (i) The free drug concentration is reduced.

   (ii) Bound drug is inactive but can act as a reservoir tending to reduce fluctuations in the concentration of free drug.

   (iii) Bound drug does not cross into the glomerular filtrate in the nephron.

   (iv) Many drugs can bind to the same site, leading to competition (see below).

PART

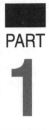

b. Drug A may displace drug B resulting in a rise in the free concentration of B and increased activity/toxicity of B. With some drugs this may be clinically important. The displaced drug would need to have been predominantly bound so that displacement of only a small proportion could cause a large increase in the free (active) drug concentration; and the displacing drug would need to occupy a large proportion of the binding sites. Thus, e.g. **sulphinpyrazone** (98% bound) may displace **warfarin** (99% bound) and markedly increase its anticoagulant action [see 📖 pp. 72–73].

10. A measure of the overall amount of a drug passing into the general circulation from the site of administration. First-pass metabolism is an important determinant of this with drugs given orally [see 📖 p. 76].

11. The volume of distribution (V_d) of a drug is the volume of fluid required to contain the total amount of the drug in the body at the same concentration as that observed in the plasma. Its magnitude is determined by the extent to which the drug is able to cross cell membranes and bind to tissue components [see 📖 pp. 80–82].

12. Plasma, fat, interstitial fluid, intracellular fluid and transcellular fluid [see 📖 p. 82 box].

13. **a.** Phase I reactions involve the oxidation, reduction or hydrolysis of drugs which in general provide the drug with a reactive group (a handle, as it were) which facilitates the phase II conjugation reactions.

   b. Phase I products are often reactive (and sometimes toxic). Phase II conjugates are generally inactive, and also readily excreted.

   [See 📖 p. 87 box.]

14. A mixed function oxidase system critical for phase I oxidation reactions [see 📖 p. 96 box].

15. Accelerated hepatic drug metabolism [see 📖 pp. 85–86, 87 box].

16. The metabolism of a drug by the gut mucosa or the liver during its passage from the intestine to the systemic circulation.

17. Glomerular filtration, passive reabsorption and tubular secretion [see 📖 p. 87].

18. **a.** Molecular size, plasma protein binding.

   b. Its lipid solubility (its state of ionisation will be relevant; see 5, 6, 7 above) or—for polar compounds—the presence of an active transport system for reabsorption, though it is uncommon for drugs to be actively reabsorbed [see 📖 pp. 87–89].

19. The volume of plasma containing the amount of substance removed by the kidney in unit time [see 📖 p. 89].

20. A drug excreted in the bile may be reabsorbed in the gastrointestinal tract and recycled, through the bloodstream to the liver, back into the gastrointestinal tract, where it may be reabsorbed … and so on. If a significant proportion of the drug undergoes this recycling, the half-life (see below) can be substantially increased.

21. When a drug which undergoes first-order elimination is given repeatedly at a constant dose, a steady-state (plateau) concentration will be reached. At this concentration the rate of elimination matches the rate of drug administration. The size of the dose and the dosing interval will determine the height of this plateau but will not have much effect on the rate at which the plasma steady-state concentration is reached. For drugs which follow saturation (zero-order) kinetics the outcome is less predictable [see 📖 p. 95, Fig. 4.25].

22. **a.** The half-life is the time taken for the plasma concentration to fall by 50%. It is directly proportional to V_d (see Answer 11

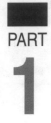

above) and inversely related to clearance in simple cases. The relevant equations are:

$t_{1/2} = 0.693/k_{el}$ where k_{el} is the elimination rate constant, and $k_{el} = CL_s/V_d$ where CL_s denotes the systemic clearance

[see 📖 pp. 91, 96 box].

b. It is clinically useful to know the $t_{1/2}$ of drugs whose elimination follows *first-order kinetics*, because the $t_{1/2}$ gives information about the duration of action and thus determines the frequency of administration. Furthermore, the time taken to reach the steady-state plasma concentration is a function of the $t_{1/2}$. In general, for repeated administration of such drugs, the amount of drug in the body will be constant and the plasma concentration will reach a plateau after about three to four half-lives.

23. The steady-state concentration of a drug is reached at a rate determined by the elimination rate constant for the drug. Accordingly, drugs with a long half-life will only achieve their plateau concentration very slowly. If a therapeutic effect is required quickly, priming or loading doses can be given to raise the plasma concentration rapidly. A safe maintenance dose rate must then be instituted, however, before toxic effects ensue.

24. Saturation kinetics: the disappearance from the plasma at a constant rate that is independent of the drug's concentration in the plasma. For drugs whose elimination follows saturation kinetics there is an unpredictable relationship between the dose and the steady-state plasma concentration on repeated application. The duration of action is strongly dependent on the dose. Such drugs are likely to cumulate [see 📖 pp. 94–96, 601–603, Fig. 30.3].

25. Yes, the plasma steady-state concentration will be reduced because the $t_{1/2}$ (which will be affected by the increased rate of metabolism) will be

reduced. To reach the original plateau the dose would have to be increased; the time taken would be three to four times the new $t_{1/2}$.

5

Chemical transmission and the autonomic nervous system

BACKGROUND INFORMATION

The autonomic nervous system regulates smooth muscle tone, exocrine and some endocrine secretions, cardiac function and has actions on intermediate metabolism. An autonomic pathway consists of two neurons: a pre- and a postganglionic neuron, with the synapse in the autonomic ganglion.

The autonomic nervous system has two main divisions, the parasympathetic and sympathetic. The enteric nervous system of the gut is a third division closely related to the former two.

The cell bodies of sympathetic preganglionic neurons are found in the lumbar and thoracic spinal cord. The preganglionic nerve fibres synapse with postganglionic neurons either just outside the spinal cord, in the paravertebral chain, or in the midline ganglia. The postganglionic fibres from the sympathetic chain join the spinal nerves. Sympathetic preganglionic fibres branch and synapse with postganglionic neurons in several segments above and below their origin in the spinal cord—an anatomical basis for a diffuse response. The para-sympathetic preganglionic fibres arise in cranial and sacral regions of the spinal cord. In contrast to their sympathetic counterparts, parasympathetic ganglia lie close to the target sites and the postganglionic fibres are usually within the tissue of the target organ. Most parasympathetic preganglionic fibres connect with only a few postganglionic fibres—an anatomical basis for discrete, localised responses.

The enteric nervous system consists of neurons with cell bodies in the plexuses in the intestinal wall. Autonomic nerves terminate on these cells but the system can operate autonomously.

The two main neurotransmitters in the autonomic nervous system are **acetylcholine** and **noradrenaline**; released from postganglionic parasympathetic and sympathetic neurons respectively. All preganglionic neurons and somatic motor nerves release acetylcholine. NANC (non-adrenergic, non-cholinergic) transmitters occur in enteric neurons, sensory neurons and as co-transmitters with noradrenaline and acetylcholine in autonomic nerves; examples include **ATP, GABA, dopamine, NO** and **peptides** (e.g. VIP). Presynaptic, autoreceptor and postsynaptic interactions between these transmitters and modulators are important.

QUESTIONS

1. Name the one part of the efferent peripheral nervous system which is not part of the autonomic nervous system.

2. **a.** Name the transmitter at the following sites:

   (i) motor nerve endings on skeletal muscle

   (ii) preganglionic sympathetic nerve terminals

   (iii) postganglionic sympathetic nerve terminals

   (iv) preganglionic parasympathetic nerve terminals

   (v) postganglionic parasympathetic nerve terminals.

   b. What is the main postsynaptic receptor at each of sites: i, ii, iv?

3. What constitutes the paravertebral chain?

4. What branch of the autonomic nervous system constitutes the cranial outflow?

5. Where are the cell bodies of the enteric nervous system located?

6. What is the main mechanism underlying presynaptic inhibition?

7. **a.** Give two examples of tissue innervated by sympathetic but not parasympathetic nerves.

b. Give two examples where the opposite applies.

8. Give three explanations of denervation supersensitivity, the general phenomenon where section of a nerve supply increases sensitivity of the target tissue.

9. What is Dale's principle of transmitter release from neurons?

10. **a.** What autoreceptors are responsible for feedback inhibition on noradrenergic and parasympathetic cholinergic nerve endings?

   b. Name some other transmitter receptor on noradrenergic nerve terminals.

11. **a.** What does NANC denote?

   b. Name some NANC transmitters.

12. Give two examples of co-transmission.

13. Indicate whether the following statements are true or false. If you think a statement is false, explain why.

   A. NA, released from noradrenergic nerves, acts on an autoreceptor to inhibit its own release.

   B. ACh, released from cholinergic nerves in cardiac tissue, stimulates NA release from adrenergic nerves.

   C. In noradrenergic nerves, an antagonist of NA, acting at the receptor mediating autoinhibitory feedback, would decrease NA release.

   D. VIP (vasoactive intestinal peptide), a co-transmitter with ACh in cholinergic nerves to salivary glands, causes vasodilatation when released.

   E. Neuropeptide Y (NPY), a co-transmitter with NA in many postganglionic noradrenergic neurons, is a vasodilator which modulates and counteracts NA-mediated vasoconstriction.

   F. Bronchial smooth muscle does not have sympathetic innervation.

   G. VIP, believed to be a co-transmitter with ACh in cholinergic nerves to

bronchial smooth muscle, reinforces the bronchoconstrictor action of ACh.

14. **a.** What would be the effect on the pupils of the eyes and the skin of the face, if postganglionic sympathetic fibres in the sympathetic chain on one side of the neck were damaged beyond repair?

   b. What would be the effect on the pupils and the facial skin, if, several weeks later, the subject were to be given an injection of adrenaline to treat an anaphylactic episode?

ANSWERS

1. The motor control of skeletal muscle [see 📖 p. 104, Fig. 5.2].

2. **a.** (i) **acetylcholine**, (ii) **acetylcholine**, (iii) **noradrenaline** (except for acetylcholine at sweat glands), (iv) **acetylcholine**, (v) **acetylcholine**.

   b. Nicotinic [see 📖 p. 104, Fig. 5.2].

3. The interconnected sympathetic ganglia which lie on either side of the spine [see 📖 p. 103, Fig. 5.1].

4. The parasympathetic system [see 📖 p. 103, Fig. 5.1]. The parasympathetic also has a sacral outflow.

5. In the intramural plexuses in the wall of the intestine [see 📖 p. 105, Fig. 5.3, p. 107 box].

6. Inhibition of the calcium entry into the nerve ending which normally follows the arrival of the action potential.

7. **a.** You could have chosen from: sweat glands, pilomotor muscles, many blood vessels, ventricular heart muscle, kidney, liver [see 📖 p. 106, Table 5.1].

   b. Ciliary muscle in the eye, bronchial smooth muscle, GIT glands, lacrimal glands [see 📖 p. 106, Table 5.1].

8. Receptor proliferation, loss of mechanism for transmitter removal and increased postsynaptic sensitivity (see 📖 pp. 107–108].

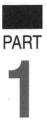

PART

1

9. That a neuron uses the same transmitter at all of its synapses. In spite of the fact that many neurons can release more than one transmitter, this principle still holds. The release of more than one transmitter at the same terminal is not precluded by the law, and there is no evidence that an individual neuron releases different transmitters at different terminals [see 📖 p. 108].

10. **a.** Alpha-2 on noradrenergic, and muscarinic (M_2) on cholinergic nerves [see 📖 p. 110, Fig. 5.5, Chs 6, 7].

b. 5-HT, ACh, adenosine, prostaglandin E_2, histamine H_2, opioid, and dopamine receptors inhibit NA release. β_2-adrenoceptors and angiotensin II receptors enhance NA release [see 📖 p. 110, Fig. 5.5, p. 111 box].

11. **a.** Non-adrenergic, non-cholinergic transmission.

b. ATP, VIP, GnRH, NPY, GABA, 5-HT, substance P, dopamine [see 📖 p. 112, Table 5.2].

12. Noradrenaline and NPY on blood vessels, where the former constricts and the latter enhances the effect by unknown mechanisms. Relatively more NPY than noradrenaline is released with higher frequency stimulation of the nerve supply. Acetylcholine and VIP in the salivary gland, where the former causes secretion and the latter vasodilates the vessels and enhances the actions of acetylcholine. Some other examples are GnRH with acetylcholine, substance P with acetylcholine [see 📖 pp. 111–113, Table 5.2, p. 113, Fig. 5.8]. It is becoming increasingly evident that co-transmission in the autonomic nervous system is important.

13. **A.** True [see 📖 p. 110, Fig. 5.5].

B. False; ACh inhibits NA release [see 📖 p. 110, Fig. 5.5].

C. False; it would increase NA release by *inhibiting* NA-mediated *inhibition* of its own release.

D. True; it is believed to increase blood flow to the glands and thus facilitate the secretory activity stimulated by ACh.

E. False; NPY enhances NA-mediated constriction [see 📖 p. 111, Fig. 5.6].

F. True, surprisingly. It has parasympathetic innervation which mediates constriction, but no sympathetic innervation. It does have a rich supply of β-receptors which respond to circulating adrenaline to give bronchodilatation [see 📖 Ch. 17].

G. False; VIP may well be a co-transmitter with ACh in the lung, but it is a bronchodilator (see 📖 Ch. 17].

14. **a.** The pupil on the damaged side would be smaller than the other pupil because there would be no NA release or NA action to counteract ACh-mediated constriction. There would also be loss of sweating in the facial skin on the damaged side because of the loss of control of sweat glands by noradrenergic fibres [see 📖 Fig. 5.2, p. 106, Table 5.1]. These phenomena, along with ptosis (a drooping eyelid) and some exophthalmos, comprise 'Horner's syndrome'.

b. If adrenaline were to be injected several weeks later, the pupil on the damaged side would react more than the other pupil because of denervation supersensitivity on the damaged side. This would be due mainly to the fact that the postganglionic fibres would have degenerated and there would be no uptake of adrenaline, but also probably due to increased numbers of adrenoceptors on the dilator pupillae, and increased postjunctional responsiveness [see 📖 pp. 107–108].

6

Cholinergic transmission

BACKGROUND INFORMATION

The main neurotransmitter released from cholinergic nerve fibres is **acetylcholine** (ACh). The two targets on which ACh acts are the nicotinic and muscarinic receptors.

Nicotinic receptors, which incorporate an ion channel in their structure, are found on postsynaptic membranes in autonomic ganglia and at the neuromuscular junction, where they mediate fast excitatory transmission. They are also found in the adrenal medulla where they stimulate release of catecholamines, and in the CNS.

Muscarinic receptors, which are coupled by G-proteins to enzymes or ion channels, mediate rather slower responses, taking seconds rather than milliseconds [see ✐ Fig. 2.3B]. There are three main types of muscarinic receptors:

- M_1-receptors are found on postsynaptic membranes in autonomic and enteric ganglia, on gastric parietal cells and in the CNS.
- M_2-receptors are found at cholinergic neuron synapses with cardiac tissue and on nerve terminals of both peripheral and central nervous systems.
- M_3-receptors are found on the postsynaptic cell membranes at postganglionic cholinergic neuron synapses with smooth muscle and with glands and on vascular endothelium.

There are specific antagonists for each type of muscarinic receptor.

ACh is synthesised from choline by choline acetyltransferase using acetylCoA as a source of acetyl groups. It is taken up, by active transport, into synaptic vesicles from whence it is released by exocytosis into the synaptic cleft. This is a Ca^{2+}-dependent process triggered by depolarisation of the nerve terminal by the action potential. The released ACh is hydrolysed by acetylcholinesterase back to choline which can be taken up again into the nerve terminal.

Drugs causing parasympathomimetic effects by acting on muscarinic receptors include **pilocarpine**, **bethanecol**, **carbachol**. (The last also acts on nicotinic receptors.)

Drugs which inhibit parasympathetic effects by antagonising ACh action on muscarinic receptors include **atropine**, **hyoscine**, **cyclopentolate**.

Drugs causing ganglion block by antagonising ACh action in ganglia include **trimetaphan**, and **hexamethonium**. (Nicotine stimulates ganglia; this is followed by depolarisation block.)

Drugs causing neuromuscular block include the non-depolarising blocking agents such as **tubocurarine**, **atracurium**, and the depolarising blocking agents, e.g. **suxamethonium** [see Fig. 5, p. 19]

Drugs which enhance cholinergic transmission do so by inhibiting acetylcholinesterase [see Fig. 6, p. 21]; this group includes:

- the short-acting agent: **edrophonium**
- medium-duration agents: **physostigmine**, **neostigmine**
- irreversible agents: **dyflos**, **ecothiopate** (these are rarely used now).

QUESTIONS

1. The muscarinic actions of *exogenous* **ACh** correspond in general to those of acetylcholine released from postganglionic parasympathetic nerve endings, but there are exceptions. What are they?

2. What transduction mechanisms mediate the cellular effects of **ACh** on M_1-, M_2-, M_3-receptors?

3. Explain what is meant by 'depolarisation block'. How does this differ from the non-depolarising block which occurs, e.g. at the neuromuscular junction?

4. There are several pharmacological agents which are muscarinic agonists.

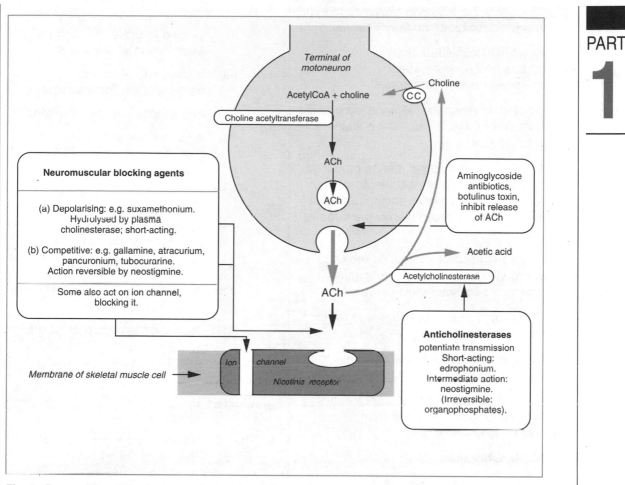

Fig. 5 Drugs acting at the neuromuscular junction. CC = choline carrier; ACh = acetylcholine. See Fig. 6 for more detail on the anticholinesterases.

What is the main clinical use of this ability to stimulate muscarinic receptors? Which drug is used? How does it act?

5. What are the main peripheral actions of atropine?

6. Which muscarinic receptor antagonists are used in the eye? What are the indications for their use?

7. What is the duration of the neuromuscular block produced by:

    a. suxamethonium, b. tubocurarine, c. pancuronium? What are the mechanisms involved in the termination of action of these agents?

8. What are the steps involved in hydrolysis of **ACh** by acetylcholinesterase?

9. How does the interaction of **neostigmine** with acetylcholinesterase differ from the interaction of **ACh** with acetylcholinesterase?

10. What will be the effects of an organophosphate insecticide (e.g. **parathion**) if it is accidentally ingested (as has happened)?

11. What is the basis for the rise in blood pressure which would occur if **carbachol** were to be injected into an experimental animal which had been given a substantial dose of **atropine**?

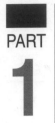

12. Where are the following enzymes found and what reactions do they catalyse:

    a. acetylcholinesterase,
    b. butyrylcholinesterase,
    c. choline acetyltransferase?

13. Indicate whether the following statements are true or false. If you think a statement is false, explain why.

    A. All the postsynaptic effects produced by **acetylcholine** at postganglionic parasympathetic nerve endings are due to action on M_3-receptors on the target organs.

    B. All **ACh** receptors outside the CNS are found on cells/tissues which are innervated by autonomic nerves.

    C. Carbachol is a selective agonist for muscarinic receptors.

    D. Suxamethonium is a depolarising neuromuscular blocking agent.

    E. Acetylcholine is the only neurotransmitter released from cholinergic nerves.

    F. Neostigmine:

    (i)   is a reversible inhibitor of acetylcholinesterase.

    (ii)   decreases gastrointestinal activity.

    (iii)   if instilled into the eye, would cause accommodation to be fixed for near vision.

    (iv)   is given orally in the treatment of myasthenia gravis.

    (v)   when used clinically is very likely to cause unwanted CNS side effects.

    (vi)   can be used to overcome the action of depolarising neuromuscular blocking agents.

    (vii)   is used i.v. in a single-dose test for the diagnosis of myasthenia gravis.

G. Atropine:

    (i)   is used to dilate the pupil for examination of the retina.

    (ii)   is used i.m. or i.v. in premedication for anaesthesia.

    (iii)   may induce urinary retention.

    (iv)   is used to overcome the bronchoconstriction of allergic asthma.

    (v)   inhibits sweating because it antagonises the action of ACh released from postganglionic parasympathetic neurons.

    (vi)   prevents motion sickness.

    (vii)   in excess doses causes serious CNS depression.

    (viii)   decreases secretion of gastric acid and spasm of gastric smooth muscle.

ANSWERS

1. The stimulation of secretion of sweat glands (which is mediated by the sympathetic system) and the release of NO from endothelium [see 📖 p. 119].

2. M_1: $InsP_3$ and DAG; M_2: decreased cyclic AMP and increased P_K or reduced P_{Ca}; M_3: $InsP_3$ and DAG [see 📖 p. 118, Table 6.1].

3. Depolarisation block involves a decrease in electrical excitability of the postsynaptic cell which occurs when the excitatory nicotinic receptors are persistently activated. The non-depolarising block which can occur at the NMJ is mainly due to competitive antagonism [see 📖 pp. 123, 133].

4. To treat glaucoma. **Pilocarpine** is the one used; being a tertiary amine it can cross the conjunctival membrane. It reduces intraocular pressure in two ways: by contracting the constrictor pupillae so that the folds of the iris do not occlude drainage of aqueous humour into the

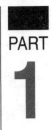

canal of Schlemm; by contracting the ciliary muscle which causes realignment of the connective tissue trabeculae through which the canal of Schlemm passes, further facilitating drainage.

5. Inhibition of secretions, tachycardia, pupillary dilatation, paralysis of accommodation, relaxation of smooth muscle of gastrointestinal tract, bronchi, bile ducts, etc, inhibition of gastric acid secretion.

6. The short-acting agents (e.g. **cyclopentolate, tropicamide**) are used for examination of the eye, long-lasting ones (e.g. **atropine**) for iritis and after eye surgery [see 📖 p. 129 box].

7. **a. Suxamethonium**: about 3 min; hydrolysed in plasma by cholinesterase.

b. Tubocurarine: about 30 min; 70% hepatic excretion, 30% renal excretion.

c. Pancuronium: about 60 min; renal excretion 80%.

[See 📖 Table 6.6, Fig. 6.10.]

8. **Step 1**: **ACh** binds to enzyme. This involves electrostatic attraction between the quaternary nitrogen atom of choline and the *anionic* site of the enzyme, and interaction of the electrophilic carbon atom of the carbonyl group with the *esteratic* site.

Step 2: The acetyl group is transferred to the serine-OH in the esteratic site; then choline dissociates leaving an acetylated enzyme.

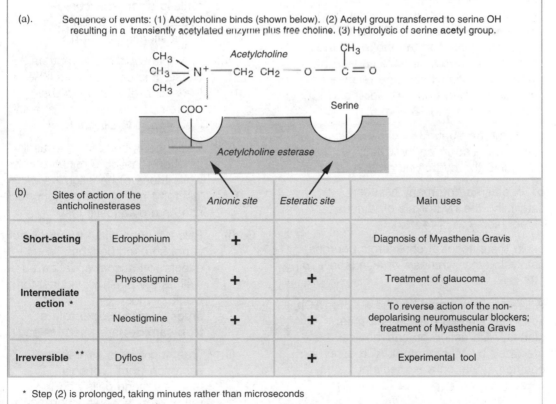

(a). Sequence of events: (1) Acetylcholine binds (shown below). (2) Acetyl group transferred to serine OH resulting in a transiently acetylated enzyme plus free choline. (3) Hydrolysis of serine acetyl group.

(b) Sites of action of the anticholinesterases		Anionic site	Esteratic site	Main uses
Short-acting	Edrophonium	+		Diagnosis of Myasthenia Gravis
Intermediate action *	Physostigmine	+	+	Treatment of glaucoma
	Neostigmine	+	+	To reverse action of the non-depolarising neuromuscular blockers; treatment of Myasthenia Gravis
Irreversible **	Dyflos		+	Experimental tool

* Step (2) is prolonged, taking minutes rather than microseconds

** The action of these agents can be reversed by pralidoxime, a reactivator of the phosphorylated enzyme. If this is used within a few hours, the covalent bond formed between the organic phosphate and the enzyme is transferred from the serine in the esteratic site to pralidoxime, leaving a functional enzyme.

Fig. 6 Cholinesterase and the anticholinesterase drugs. (a) Outline of the action of cholinesterase on acetylcholine. (b) The sites of action and main uses of the anticholinesterase drugs.

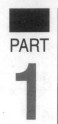

Step 3: The acetylated moiety reacts with water to give acetic acid and regenerated enzyme [see Fig. 6 and ✎ Fig. 6.12].

9. Step 3 (see above) takes minutes rather than microseconds [see ✎ p. 140].

10. The organophosphate insecticides are anticholinesterases and will produce a range of parasympathomimetic actions, such as salivation and bronchoconstriction; increased concentrations of ACh at the neuromuscular junction can produce spontaneous twitching and, if excessive, depolarisation block and paralysis; CNS stimulation may give rise to convulsions.

11. **Carbachol** stimulates the nicotinic receptors in all autonomic ganglia (both parasympathetic and sympathetic) and in the adrenal medulla; but all the parasympathetic effects would be blocked by the **atropine**. The rise in blood pressure would be due to the vasoconstriction and the inotropic and chronotropic cardiac effects caused by sympathetic stimulation and release of **catecholamines** from the adrenal medulla [see ✎ p. 118, Fig. 6.1].

12. **a.** Membrane-bound in cholinergic synapses, also in erythrocytes; catalysing the hydrolysis of ACh.

    b. In plasma and many tissues; catalysing the hydrolysis of various esters [see ✎ p. 144 box].

    c. In the cytosol of cholinergic neurons; catalysing the synthesis of ACh [see ✎ p. 124 box].

13. **A.** False. This would be true only for **ACh** action on smooth muscle and most glands. ACh action on cardiac tissue is mediated by M_2-receptors; ACh action on gastric parietal cells is mediated by M_1-receptors (see ✎ p. 118, Table 6.1).

    B. False. Vascular endothelium has muscarinic M_3-receptors, but is not innervated by autonomic nerves; the receptors are on the luminal aspect of the endothelium.

C. False. It also acts at nicotinic receptors.

D. True.

E. False. There are co-transmitters in some (if not all) cholinergic nerves [see ✎ p. 111, Table 5.2].

F. (i) True.

    (ii) False; it increases peristaltic activity and is used to treat paralytic ileus.

    (iii) True; but it is not used in the eye; physostigmine is used (in treatment of glaucoma).

    (iv) True [see ✎ p. 142, Table 6.7].

    (v) False; it is a quaternary ammonium compound and of low lipid solubility; it therefore penetrates poorly into the CNS (unless given in excessive dosage [see ✎ to compare with physostigmine p. 144].

    (vi) False; it would make matters worse. It is used to overcome the action of *non-depolarising* neuromuscular blocking agents [see ✎ p. 145 clinical box]

    (vii) False; edrophonium is so used, its effects lasting 5 minutes only, while those of neostigmine can last for 4 hours—far too long for use as a diagnostic test.

G. (i) False; it does dilate the pupil but is not so used because its effects (on accommodation as well as the pupil) would last for a week or more. Short-acting drugs (e.g. **cyclopentolate**, **tropicamide**) are used instead.

    (ii) True; it prevents the reflex secretion from bronchial mucosal gland cells and the reflex bronchoconstriction which might otherwise be triggered by irritant inhalation anaesthetics.

    (iii) True, especially in elderly patients. It inhibits **ACh-**

mediated contraction of the detrusor muscle of the bladder and relaxation of the sphincter.

(iv) False; muscarinic receptor antagonists are only used in asthma in which there is a component of parasympathetic-mediated reflex spasm and the drug then used is **ipratropium** which is used as an adjunct to other therapy [see 📖 p. 360 box].

(v) False; it does inhibit sweating, but does so by antagonising the **ACh** released from postganglionic sympathetic neurons.

(vi) True; but **hyoscine** is actually the muscarinic antagonist which is used for motion sickness [see 📖 p. 129].

(vii) False; in excess doses it causes marked CNS stimulation. **Hyoscine**, in excess amounts, causes CNS stimulation, but is sedative in normally used dosage.

(viii) True; but atropine is not the drug of choice when these actions are required clinically in patients with peptic ulcer. H_2 **antagonists** or **omeprazole** are the drugs of choice for decreasing gastric acid secretion [see 📖 pp. 389–391]. If antimuscarinic drugs are used, the M_1 antagonist, pirenzepine (reported to be effective for reduction of acid secretion) is preferred to atropine [see 📖 p. 391].

7

Noradrenergic transmission

BACKGROUND INFORMATION

CLASSIFICATION OF ADRENOCEPTORS

Early experiments of Dale and later of Ahlquist and of Lands led to the emergence of the concept of different subtypes of adrenoceptors, which are at present classified as α_1, α_2, β_1, β_2, β_3. The distinction between the presynaptic and postsynaptic receptors at the synapse of the noradrenergic neuron with target tissue should be grasped. It is also important to know the differences in the locations of the various post-synaptic receptor subtypes in different tissues, and the effects of stimulating each type of receptor in each target tissue [see 📖 Table 7.1]. Many clinically important drugs act by modifying noradrenergic transmission.

THE PHYSIOLOGY OF NORADRENERGIC TRANSMISSION

The enzymic steps in the synthesis of the transmitter, **noradrenaline** (NA), start with tyrosine (which is taken up into the neuron) and progress to DOPA and then **dopamine**, which is taken up into the storage vesicles, where it is converted to **NA**. NA content of the cytosol of the neuron is low, due to breakdown by monoamine oxidase. NA release occurs by Ca^{2+}-mediated exocytosis initiated by a nerve action potential. This process is modulated by auto-inhibitory feedback by the released NA on presynaptic α_2-receptors. Some drugs can also cause NA release. The action of the released transmitter is short-lived because there is rapid active re-uptake into the nerve terminals and from there into the storage vesicles.

In the adrenal medulla some NA is converted to adrenaline and both substances are released

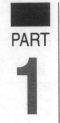

PART 1

under the influence of the relevant splanchnic nerve fibres.

Drugs acting on adrenoceptors

Because of the differences between the various adrenoceptor subtypes it has proved possible to develop drugs which act selectively, as agonists or antagonists, on these different receptors. Some are stimulants (agonists) at adrenoceptors, with varying potency and selectivity at the various subclasses of receptor. Others (antagonists) block the action of agonists, again with varying potency and selectivity at different receptor subtypes. The specificity of the effect at particular subtypes of adrenoceptor determines the overall pharmacological actions of a drug and its clinical use.

Prototype examples are:

Agonist	Antagonist
α_1: **phenylephrine**	**prazosin**
α_2: **clonidine**	**yohimbine** (experimental tool)
β_1: **isoprenaline** (also active on β_2)	**atenolol**
β_2: **salbutamol**	**propranolol** (also active on β_1) **butoxamine** (experimental tool)

Drugs acting on the noradrenergic neuron

Pharmacological agents can modify the events occurring in the noradrenergic neuron in a variety of different ways:

- by modifying noradrenaline synthesis, e.g. **carbidopa** (which inhibits it), **methyldopa** (which gives rise to a false transmitter)
- by affecting noradrenaline storage, e.g. **reserpine**
- by affecting the process of release of transmitter, e.g. noradrenergic neuron blocking drugs such as **guanethidine**
- by displacing noradrenaline from the neuron, e.g. **amphetamine**
- by acting on the presynaptic adrenoceptor, e.g. **clonidine** (attenuates release of NA)
- by inhibition of the uptake of noradrenaline, e.g. **cocaine.**

QUESTIONS

1. **a.** Give examples of drugs acting as agonists mainly on the receptors specified:

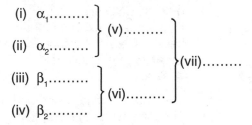

(i) α_1.........
(ii) α_2.........
(iii) β_1.........
(iv) β_2 ....
(v).........
(vi).........
(vii).........

   b. Will all of these agents result in increased sympathomimetic activity? If not, which will have the opposite effect?

2. Which α-adrenoceptor antagonist has effects which may be due to partial agonist activity?

3. **a.** Give examples of drugs acting *mainly* as antagonists on the receptors specified:

(i) α_1.........
(ii) α_2.........
(iii) β_1.........
(iv) β_2.........
(v).........
(vi).........
(vii).........

   b. Will all of these agents result in decreased sympathomimetic activity? If not, which will have the opposite effect?

   c. Are all the agents listed clinically useful?

4. **a.** Give an example of an irreversible competitive antagonist at α_1-receptors.

   b. What is the basis for the irreversibility?

   c. What other actions does this drug have?

5. **a.** List the main steps in **noradrenaline** synthesis.

   b. What drugs can interfere with this? Are they clinically useful, and if so what for?

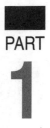

PART

1

6. a. How is **noradrenaline** held in the nerve terminal? How is it released from the nerve terminal?

b. What receptors are involved in regulating this release?

c. What drugs can inhibit the NA release mechanism? Are they clinically useful, and if so what for?

7. a. What β_2 actions are clinically useful?

b. Give an example of a drug which is a β-adrenoceptor agonist with actions on both β_1- and β_2-adrenoceptors.

c. If this drug is used therapeutically for its β_2 actions, will the β_1 effects be useful or unwanted, and if so why?

8. For what condition(s) is injection of a drug acting on adrenoceptors an emergency, life-saving measure?

9. α_1-antagonists such as **a** .... and **b**......... will reduce blood pressure by an action on **c**......... (specify receptors and tissue), but the heart rate will increase for the following reasons **d**......... **e**..........

10. a. What is the local fate of noradrenaline (NA) after release from the nerve terminal?

b. How does this differ from the fate of acetylcholine?

11. What are the main therapeutic uses of β-adrenoceptor antagonists? (These are important.)

12. a. Which drug can produce a 'chemical sympathectomy'?

b. Work out which sympathomimetic drugs would cease to act after a 'chemical sympathectomy'.

13. In an anaesthetised animal whose blood pressure is being recorded, injection of **tyramine** causes a rise in blood pressure. If the injection is repeated every 10 minutes or so, the response gradually gets less and less. What is the mechanism underlying the rise in blood pressure? What is the basis for the attenuation of the response? How could the response be restored?

14. Cocaine addicts, who take the drug by sniffing, may develop necrosis of the nasal mucous membrane. What is the basis of this effect?

15. a. Give examples of adrenoceptor stimulating drugs which are given by inhalation.

b. What condition(s) are such drugs usually used for?

16. Outline the effects on pulse rate, blood pressure, and peripheral resistance which would be produced in man by intravenous infusion of:

a. noradrenaline

b. isoprenaline

c. adrenaline.

17. What are the main differences in the priorities and actions of the β-receptor antagonists? Do these differences have clinical significance?

18. Figure 7 gives a schematic diagram of the noradrenergic neuron and a target cell. There are at least nine sites where drugs can affect the process of NA synthesis, release, uptake or action. Indicate these sites, specifying the groups of drugs which act at each site.

19. Indicate which of the following statements are true and which false. If you think a statement is false, explain why.

A. α_1-**adrenoceptor stimulants** contract vascular smooth muscle.

B. α_1-**adrenoceptor stimulants** relax non-sphincter gastrointestinal muscle.

C. α_1-**adrenoceptor stimulants** relax uterine smooth muscle.

D. The rate-limiting step in NA synthesis is that catalysed by dopa-decarboxylase.

E. The main mechanism for terminating the transmitter action of **NA** is through

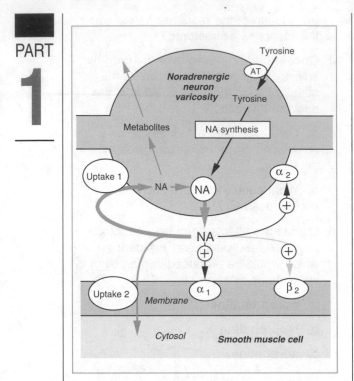

Fig. 7 Schematic diagram of the junction of sympathetic neuron with target cell. NA = noradrenaline; AT = active transport.

metabolism by monoamine oxidase and/or COMT.

F. Isoprenaline has a selective action on β_1-receptors.

G. Catecholamines promote the conversion of the body's energy stores (glycogen and fat) to freely available fuel (glucose, free fatty acids).

H. β_1-blockers are useful in hypertension because (i) they decrease cardiac output by inhibiting the inotropic and chronotropic action of NA on β_1-receptors in the heart, and (ii) they do not significantly block the vasodilator effect of endogenous adrenaline on β_2-receptors in the blood vessels.

I. Propranolol is contraindicated in patients with asthma.

J. β-adrenoceptor antagonists are contraindicated in hypertension.

K. Prazosin is an α_2-selective antagonist.

L. Phentolamine is a short-acting reversible competitive antagonist at α-receptors.

M. Non-selective α-**receptor antagonists** cause a fall in blood pressure by their blocking action at α_1-receptors, but this is offset by their α_2-blocking effect which tends to increase **NA** release with resultant inotropic and chronotropic effects on the heart. (Think about this.)

N. Adrenaline, noradrenaline, isoprenaline, salbutamol are all catecholamines.

O. The β_2-adrenoceptor antagonist, **salbutamol**, has potent bronchodilator properties and is effective therapy for asthmatic bronchospasm.

P. Carbidopa inhibits DOPA decarboxylase, thus decreasing NA synthesis; it can therefore prevent peripheral effects of **L-dopa** (used to treat Parkinsonism) which result from conversion of L-dopa to dopamine and noradrenaline.

Q. Guanethidine, a noradrenergic neuron blocker, is taken up into noradrenergic neuron varicosities by uptake 2, and stored in synaptic vesicles.

R. Methyldopa gives rise to a false transmitter (methyl-NA) which has potent action on the presynaptic α_2-receptors thus reducing NA release. It can thus reduce blood pressure.

ANSWERS

1. a. Some examples are:

(i) **methoxamine, phenylephrine, oxymetazoline**

(ii) **clonidine**

(iii) **dobutamine**

(iv) **salbutamol, terbutaline**

(v) **isoprenaline**

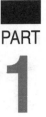

PART

1

(vi) **noradrenaline**

(vii) **adrenaline**

[see 📖 p. 162 box, Table 7.2].

b. All will have some; some will have all the effects of sympathetic stimulation, with the exception of **clonidine**, an α_2-agonist, which will decrease NA release.

2. **Ergotamine** [see 📖 Table 7.2].

3. **a.** Some examples are:

(i) **prazosin, indoramin**

(ii) **yohimbine**

(iii) **atenolol**

(iv) **butoxamine**

(v) **phenoxybenzamine, phentolamine**

(vi) **propranolol, oxprenolol**

(vii) **labetalol**

[see 📖 Table 7.2]. Note that not all the above agents are totally selective for the receptors specified.

b. Yohimbine, an α_2-antagonist, will inhibit the auto-inhibitory feedback of NA and thus *increase* NA release.

c. Yohimbine is an experimental tool and is not used clinically.

4. **a. Phenoxybenzamine**.

b. It binds covalently to the receptor.

c. It is an antagonist at α_2-receptors and blocks uptake 1 (and 2). It also antagonises the actions of ACh, histamine and 5-HT [see 📖 p. 163, Table 7.3].

5. **a.** L-tyrosine → DOPA → dopamine → NA [see 📖 p. 158 box].

b. See Answer 32, page 169, and Figure 32, page 170; also 📖 Table 7.4.

6. **a.** NA is held in synaptic vesicles along with ATP, chromogranin and dopamine β-hydroxylase. The action potential induced depolarisation opens Ca^{2+} channels and NA is released by Ca^{2+}-mediated exocytosis. (Some drugs can displace NA from the vesicles into the cytoplasm from where it may pass into the synaptic cleft by carrier-mediated diffusion) [see 📖 Fig. 7.11].

b. Presynaptic α_2-receptors inhibit NA release (ACh and prostaglandins also inhibit release).

c. Noradrenergic neuron blockers (e.g. **guanethidine**); used for hypertension [see 📖 Figs 5.5, 5.10, 7.4, 7.11, Table 7.4, p. 158 box].

7. **a.** The main clinically desirable β_2 actions are bronchodilatation in asthma and uterine relaxation in premature labour.

b. Isoprenaline [see 📖 Table 7.2].

c. β_1 actions on the heart will be unwanted.

8. Subcutaneous **adrenaline** can be life-saving in acute anaphylactic shock. (**Dobutamine**, and possibly **dopamine**, may have a role in the treatment of cardiogenic shock. α_1-agonists such as **methoxamine** have been used in atrial tachycardia, but cardioversion or the use of antidysrhythmic drugs [see 📖 Ch. 13] are generally safer.)

9. **a. phenoxybenzamine; b. phentolamine; c.** α_1-receptors on arterial muscle. **d.** These drugs also inhibit α_2-receptors thus decreasing the negative feedback of NA on its own release, and this α_2-inhibition on noradrenergic neurons to the heart means more NA is released to act on β_1-receptors, which **e** are not inhibited by the two drugs [see 📖 p. 163].

10. **a.** It is taken up again into the noradrenergic neuron by uptake 1 and into other tissues by uptake 2 [see Fig. 8 and 📖 Table 7.3].

b. Acetylcholine is not taken up; it is hydrolysed in the synaptic space [see 📖 pp. 124 box, 144 box].

PART

1

11. Important uses:

hypertension, cardiac dysrhythmias, angina pectoris, myocardial infarction.

They are also used for glaucoma, anxiety states, and as adjuncts to the therapy of hyperthyroidism [see 📖 p. 166 clinical box].

12. a. 6-hydroxydopamine.

b. All drugs which are sympathomimetic by action on the sympathetic neuron, e.g. indirectly acting sympathomimetic agents and those that increase sympathetic action through prolonging the action of the transmitter by inhibiting uptake of NA [see 📖 Table 7.4].

13. Tyramine causes an increase in blood pressure by releasing NA from noradrenergic neuron varicosities. The response decreases (this is called 'tachyphylaxis') because the store of NA decreases; i.v. injection of NA will replenish the stores and restore the response [see 📖 p. 155].

14. The block of uptake leads to increased local NA, therefore sustained, increased local α_1-mediated vasoconstriction [see 📖 Tables 7.1, 7.3].

15. a. β_2-agonists such as **salbutamol** and **terbutaline**.

b. Asthma [see 📖 Table 7.4].

16. a. **Noradrenaline** increases the systolic and diastolic pressure and the peripheral resistance (β_1 inotropic action plus α_1 vasoconstriction) but decreases heart rate (baroreceptor reflex).

b. **Isoprenaline** reduces peripheral resistance (β_2 vasodilatation), increases heart rate (β_1 chronotropic effect + reflex tachycardia), but diastolic pressure is reduced (β_2 vasodilatation) and systolic minimally increased (β_1 inotropic action).

c. **Adrenaline** increases heart rate (β_1 effect), increases systolic pressure (β_1) decreases diastolic pressure (β_2 vaso-dilatation) and decreases peripheral resistance (β_2 vasodilatation). [See 📖 Fig. 7.8.]

17. The β-adrenoceptor antagonists can differ in several respects including (i) their selectivity for β_1- over β_2-receptors, (ii) their partial agonist activity, (iii) their solubility in lipid or water, (iv) their half-lives, (v) their metabolism and (vi) their putative propensity to lead to increased plasma triglycerides and reduced HDL cholesterol. There are also some differences in routes of administration.

Blockers with predominantly β_1 actions (e.g. **metoprolol**, **atenolol**) are cardioselective (though they all have some β_2-blocking action). Agents which are water-soluble (e.g. **atenolol**) are less likely to enter the CNS and are therefore less likely to cause nightmares and sleeplessness; furthermore, being excreted in the urine, they could cumulate in renal insufficiency. Agents with partial agonist activity (e.g. **oxprenolol**) are less likely to cause bradycardia and cold hands and feet, and may also be less likely to increase serum triglycerides since they will have some stimulant action on β_1-receptor-mediated stimulation of the fat cell hormone-sensitive lipase which catalyses breakdown of triglycerides [see 📖 Fig. 15.1, Table 7.1].

The action on β_2-receptors of endogenous **adrenaline** and β_2-agonists such as **salbutamol** is important in asthma; thus β-blockers which block β_2-receptors can cause serious problems if used in asthmatic patients. **Adrenaline**, by action on β_2-receptors increases glycogenolysis, thus promoting hyperglycaemia and functioning as a counter-regulatory hormone to insulin [see 📖 Table 20.2]; therefore, β-blockers which block β_2-receptors could compromise the recovery of insulin-dependent diabetics from episodes of hypoglycaemia. In these patients, if β-block is required, a β_1-selective blocker would be safer.

As regards routes of administration, all can be given orally (though **metoprolol**

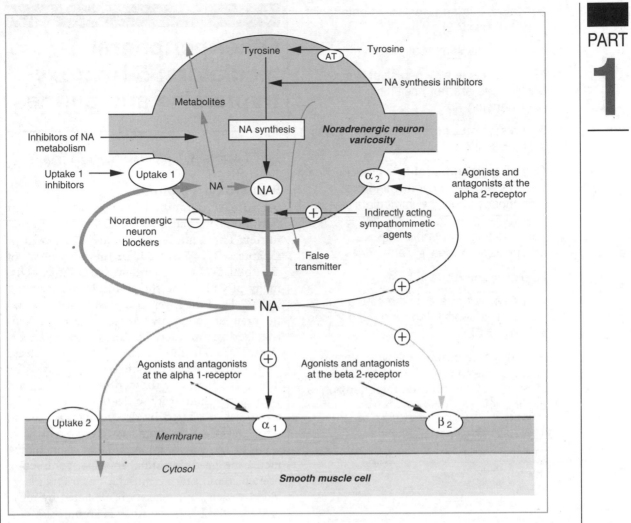

Fig. 8 Drugs affecting noradrenaline (NA) synthesis, release and action at the junction of sympathetic neuron with target cell. AT = active transport.

and **propranolol** are *subject to significant first-pass metabolism*) and **atenolol**, **propranolol**, **metoprolol** and **labetalol** can also be given i.v.

18. See Figure 8. Note NA has very little action on β_2-receptors. More detail on these drugs is given in Figure 32 [see also 📖 Fig. 7.12].

19. A. True [see 📖 Table 7.1].

B. True [see 📖 p. 159].

C. False; α_1-agonists contract the uterus; β_2-stimulants relax it [see 📖 Table 7.1].

D. False; it is the step catalysed by tyrosine hydroxylase (see 📖 Fig. 7.3].

E. False; it is by rapid, active transport re-uptake into the neuronal varicosity [see 📖 p. 155].

F. False; it is active on both β_1- and β_2-receptors [see 📖 Table 7.2].

G. True [see 📖 p. 160].

H. True [see 📖 p. 265].

I. True; it would prevent the necessary β_2-mediated bronchodilator action of endogenous adrenaline [see 📖 p. 166].

J. False; they are first-line drugs for hypertension treatment [see 📖 p. 166 box and Table 7.4].

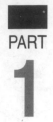

K. False; it is an α_1-selective antagonist [see ▱ Table 7.2].

L. True [see ▱ p. 163].

M. True; this is why non-selective α-antagonists are not useful in hypertension.

N. False; **salbutamol** is not [see ▱ Fig. 7.1 and p. 174].

O. False; **salbutamol** is a bronchodilator and is effective in overcoming the bronchospasm in the immediate phase of asthma [see ▱ Ch. 17], but this is because it is an *agonist* at β_2-adrenoceptors [see ▱ Table 7.4].

P. True [see ▱ p. 167].

Q. False; but true if, in the statement, uptake 1 is substituted for uptake 2 [see ▱ Table 7.3].

R. True; but its main antihypertensive effect is due to an action in the CNS. (The use of this drug for hypertension is declining.)

8

Other peripheral mediators: 5-hydroxy-tryptamine and purines

BACKGROUND INFORMATION

5-Hydroxytryptamine

5-Hydroxytryptamine (5-HT) is an important peripheral mediator and central neurotransmitter. The central actions are dealt with in Chapters 24, 27 and 29. In the body, 90% of the total 5-HT is found in chromaffin cells, many of which line the stomach and intestine wall. Cells of the myenteric plexus, platelets and the brain are other major sources. 5-HT is synthesised from tryptophan via 5-hydroxytryptophan. The mechanisms for storage, release and re-uptake are similar to those for noradrenaline, and these processes, together with monoamine oxidase degradation of 5-HT, are therefore altered by drugs which act at the same stages on the noradrenaline system.

5-HT has several important actions including increasing gastrointestinal motility, contracting bronchial and uterine muscle, constricting large blood vessels (but relaxation mediated by nitric oxide synthesis can occur—via stimulation of a different 5-HT receptor), dilating small arterioles and constricting small venules. Platelet aggregation and stimulation of nociceptors are also important actions. There are many subtypes of 5-HT receptors, the classification of which is still evolving. In the current classification, 5-HT_1 receptors (A, B, D varieties) produce effects via inhibition of adenylate cyclase, whereas 5-HT_4 receptors stimulate adenylate cyclase. 5-HT_2 receptors (A, B, C varieties) activate PLC. 5-HT_3 receptors have an integral ion channel (like nicotinic receptors) [see ▱ Table 8.1, p.182 box]. Migraine and the carcinoid syndrome are clinical conditions where treatment with drugs affecting 5-HT receptors is important.

Purines

The purines, adenosine, ADP and ATP, produce pharmacological effects independently of their role in energy metabolism. ATP is now recognised to act as both a neurotransmitter and co-transmitter. It acts on P_2-receptors which are divided into P_{2X}-receptors, which possess an integral ion channel, and P_{2Y}-receptors, which couple to G-proteins. Adenosine has its own receptors, A_1 and A_2, but the full details of its synthesis and release remain unclear. It may function as a mediator in the CNS and as a local regulator of vascular and bronchial smooth muscle.

Drugs which act on 5-HT receptors and which are used clinically include **ondansetron, methysergide, cyproheptadine**. A drug which acts on purine receptors, and which is used clinically, is **theophylline**.

QUESTIONS

1. Name three sites where high levels of 5-HT are found.

2. **a.** What is the specific enzyme for 5-HT synthesis?

   b. What enzymes are responsible for the degradation of 5-HT and what is the final product?

3. What is the action of 5-HT on the intestine?

4. What stimulates 5-HT release from chromaffin cells?

5. Name four actions of 5-HT on the vasculature.

6. What effect does 5-HT have on platelets?

7. Which 5-HT receptor mediates inhibitory effects on neurons?

8. Which 5-HT receptor is involved in pain transmission?

9. What is the clinical action of **a. ondansetron b. sumatriptan**? What are their therapeutic effects?

10. Which is the autoreceptor for 5-HT (i.e. the one which modifies the neuronal release of 5-HT)?

11. **a.** Describe the main effects of adenosine.

b. Adenosine could be implicated in the pathogenesis of two important clinical conditions. What are they?

12. Indicate whether the following statements are true or false. If you think a statement is false, explain why.

A. Most 5-HT is located in the CNS.

B. The 5-HT receptor found on vascular smooth muscle is the 5-HT_1 type.

C. An antagonist of the 5-HT_3 receptor is a very useful anti-emetic drug.

D. Platelets actively take up 5-HT as they pass through the intestinal circulation.

E. 5-HT is stored, in substantial amounts, in human mast cells, along with histamine.

F. **Methysergide** is an antagonist at 5-HT_{2C} receptors.

G. Ergotamine is a partial agonist at 5-HT_1 receptors

H. 5-HT is released from platelets at sites of tissue damage.

I. **Ketanserin,** a 5-HT_2 receptor antagonist, blocks the vasodilator effects of 5-HT.

J. 5-HT has an inhibitory effect on the enteric neurons.

K. Both 5-HT agonists and antagonists can be useful in migraine.

L. Carcinoid syndrome is characterised by the release from enterochromaffin tumour cells of 5-HT, substance P, prostaglandins, and bradykinin—5-HT being the most important.

M. A 5-HT_3 antagonist can control many of the symptoms of carcinoid syndrome.

N. **Somatostatin** is useful in treatment of carcinoid syndrome because it antagonises 5-HT actions.

O. ATP is contained in the synaptic vesicles of both noradrenergic and cholinergic neurons.

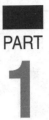

PART

1

PART

1

P. ATP is released from noradrenergic nerves as a co-transmitter with noradrenaline.

Q. The effects of the purine, adenosine, are mediated by two separate receptors, P_1 and P_2.

R. The effects of ATP are mediated by A_1- and A_2-receptors.

S. ATP is responsible for the slow synaptic responses.

T. ATP released from purinergic nerves causes the opening of K^+ channels in the target cell membrane.

U. Theophylline is an antagonist at the adenosine A_1-receptor.

ANSWERS

1. The gut wall, platelets and the brain [see 🗐 p. 177].

2. **a.** Tryptophan hydroxylase.

   b. Monoamine oxidase and aldehyde dehydrogenase metabolise 5-HT to 5-hydroxyindoleacetic acid (5-HIAA) [see 🗐 Fig. 8.1].

3. It increases motility, partly by acting directly on the smooth muscle and partly via enteric neurons. The peristaltic reflex involves the release of 5-HT from chromaffin cells by the mechanical stimulus of food in the lumen [see 🗐 p. 178].

4. Vagal stimulation [see 🗐 p. 178].

5. **a.** Inhibition of **noradrenaline** release (reducing vasoconstrictor tone).

   b. Dilatation of precapillary vessels by releasing NO from endothelial cells [see 🗐 Ch. 14].

   c. Increased capillary permeability.

   d. Constriction of postcapillary vessels by a direct action on smooth muscle. Thus dilatation and fluid leakage result [see 🗐 Fig. 8.3].

6. It causes aggregation [see 🗐 pp. 179–180].

7. 5-HT_1, types A and B [see 🗐 Table 8.1].

8. The 5-HT_3 receptor, which is found on nociceptive sensory neurons [see 🗐 Table 8.1].

9. **a.** 5-HT_3 antagonist.

   b. 5-HT_{1D} agonist.

   Ondansetron is an anti-emetic; **sumatriptan** has anti-migraine activity. [See 🗐 p. 182, 187 box.]

10. The 5-HT_1 receptor [see 🗐 Table 8.1].

11. **a.** Effects at A_1-receptors: block of AV conduction, bronchoconstriction and inhibition of transmitter release in CNS and PNS, vasoconstriction in the kidney. Effects at A_2-receptors: vasodilatation, inhibition of platelet aggregation, stimulation of cardiac nociceptors [see 🗐 p. 189].

    b. It may be implicated in anginal pain and may contribute to broncho-constriction in asthmatic subjects [see 🗐 p. 189].

12. **A.** False; 90% of the total 5-HT in the body occurs in the chromaffin cells in the GIT [see 🗐 p. 177].

    B. False; it is 5-HT_2 [see 🗐 Table 8.1].

    C. True; **ondansetron** is proving to be very useful clinically [see 🗐 p. 182, Fig. 19.8, p. 396].

    D. True [see 🗐 pp. 177–178].

    E. False; 5-HT is stored in mast cells in rodents, but there is little or no 5-HT in human mast cells.

    F. True [see 🗐 Table 8.1].

    G. True; [see 🗐 Table 8.1].

    H. True [see 🗐 p. 177].

    I. False; **ketanserin** is a 5-HT_2 receptor antagonist but it blocks the direct vasoconstrictor effects of 5-HT on vascular smooth muscle [see 🗐 Fig. 8.2].

J. False; it has an excitatory effect [see 📖 p. 178].

K. Surprisingly, this is true, the drugs being:

sumatriptan (5-HT$_1$ agonist),

ergotamine (5-HT$_1$ partial agonist),

methysergide, **cyproheptadine** (5-HT$_2$ antagonists).

L. True [see 📖 p. 186].

M. False; this statement applies to the 5-HT$_2$ antagonist, **cyproheptadine** (this drug also displays H$_1$-receptor antagonism) [see 📖 pp. 187, 261].

N. False; somatostatin may be of value, but the reason is that it suppresses the secretion of the relevant mediators [see 📖 p. 187].

O. True [see 📖 p. 187].

P. True [see 📖 p. 187].

Q. False; the receptors are termed A$_1$ and A$_2$ [see 📖 p. 187].

R. False; ATP receptors are termed P$_2$-receptors (adenosine receptors were originally referred to as P$_1$-receptors) [see 📖 p. 188].

S. False; acting on ligand-gated ion channels it is responsible for the fast synaptic responses [see 📖 p. 189 box].

T. True; ATP, acting on P$_{2Y}$-receptors can increase [Ca^{2+}] in smooth muscle, which, in turn, can activate Ca^{2+}-dependent K$^+$ channels. (This action should be distinguished from the action of intracellular ATP to inhibit K$_{ATP}$ channels in cardiac muscle and pancreatic β-cells.)

U. True [see 📖 p. 188].

9

Peptides as mediators

BACKGROUND INFORMATION

Peptides are now known to be important as neurotransmitters/mediators in many physiological and pathological reactions. Most known, pharmacologically-active peptides are found in the nervous system or in endocrine glands, but some are derived from the plasma, the cells of the immune system, the vascular endothelium, etc. The number of peptides with roles in the regulation of bodily function now greatly exceeds that of non-peptides. Peptides are chains of amino acids, containing up to 50 amino-acid residues, above which the term 'protein' is used. Pharmacologically active peptides are derived from large, inactive, precursor proteins. There are many sequence similarities between different active peptides and considerable diversity can arise from differences in the processing of the precursor.

The mechanisms involved in the release or generation vary with the site and function of the peptides. The release of a peptide hormone may be stimulated by another hormone (e.g. CRF regulates ACTH release) [see 📖 Fig. 21.13]. Peptides derived from precursors in the plasma may be generated by enzyme action in the plasma (e.g. angiotensin I by renin action) [see 📖 Fig. 14.5]. Some peptides, particularly the co-transmitters (such as vasoactive intestinal peptide which occurs in some parasympathetic nerves) [see 📖 Table 5.2], are released by the nerve action potential. The release, binding and actions of peptide neurotransmitters can be similar to those of the classic transmitters. However, there is no uptake on release; instead peptides are cleaved by peptidases to inactive products.

Analogues and antagonists are being developed as well as preparations of endogenous peptides, but progress is hampered by the fact

PART

1

that drugs based on peptides are often poorly absorbed, and may be rapidly degraded, while those destined for action in the CNS do not easily cross the blood–brain barrier. In certain cases many of these problems have been circumvented [see 📖 Table 9.2]. In the case of the endogenous opioids, non-peptide agonists and antagonists are available.

- Important peptide mediators: **bradykinin, opioid peptides, tachykinins, angiotensin II**.
- Clinically useful peptide drugs include: **oxytocin, vasopressin, cyclosporin** [see 📖 Table 9.2).

QUESTIONS

1. Can more than one active peptide arise from a single precursor prohormone?

2. Name two pharmacologically active peptides derived from plasma proteins.

3. Which peptides are known to have receptors directly linked to ion channels?

4. Give an example of two peptides which are co-transmitters, i.e. peptides which are held in, and released from the same neuron as a classic transmitter.

5. A single precursor gene may give rise to several peptides. Give an example of two pharmacologically active peptides which are coded for by the same gene.

6. **a.** ...., a member of the group of peptides termed **b.** .... is released at the central terminals of nociceptive neurons and is thought to serve as a transmitter of pain. **c.** .... is a potent vasoconstrictor peptide derived from vascular endothelial cells.

7. Give examples of drugs, interacting with peptide receptors, which are not themselves peptides.

8. What peptides are derived from preproopiomelanocortin (POMC)?

9. **Met-enkephalin** and **β-endorphin** are both opioid peptides. The five amino acids which comprise met-enkephalin

occur within β-endorphin. Are these two peptides coded for by the same gene or different genes?

10. What are the three opioid receptors?

11. Name three tachykinins.

12. Some tachykinins are found in some peripheral sensory neurons. Which are these neurons and what happens following release of the tachykinins at: **a.** the central endings; **b.** the peripheral endings of these neurons?

13. Name four peptides for which competitive antagonists are known.

ANSWERS

1. Yes, two or even more can be produced [see 📖 p. 196 box, Fig. 9.3].

2. **Bradykinin** and **angiotensin II**, both important targets for therapy [see 📖 pp. 239, 313]. Other important peptides derived from plasma are the **complement components** [see 📖 Fig. 11.1].

3. None. Although release of peptides can be fast, synthesis is slow, so linkage to a rapid effector system would not really make biological sense.

4. **Vasoactive intestinal polypeptide** (VIP) with **acetylcholine** in the parasympathetic supply to the salivary gland; **neuropeptide Y** with **noradrenaline** in the sympathetic supply to many blood vessels; **cholecystokinin** with **dopamine** in the nucleus accumbens [see 📖 Ch. 28, p. 193, also Table 5.2].

5. **Calcitonin/CGRP**, and **substance P/ substance K** (also known as neurokinin A) are examples of peptide pairs produced from the same gene by differences in splicing [see 📖 p. 236].

6. **a. Substance P, b. tachykinins, c. endothelin** [see 📖 pp. 199–200].

7. Morphine and related drugs acting on opioid receptors; losartan on angiotensin receptors and lorglumide on cholecystokinin receptors [see ✎ Table 9.1].

8. **Endorphin**, **ACTH** and **MSH** [see ✎ Fig. 9.3].

9. They are coded for by different genes [see ✎ p. 199].

10. μ, δ, and κ [see ✎ p. 199, also Ch. 31].

11. The main ones which are important in humans are **substance P**, **neurokinin A** (also known as substance K) and **neurokinin B**. There are others in amphibians and in the octopus [see ✎ pp. 199–200].

12. The nociceptive neurons are the sensory neurons which contain tachykinins.

    a. Release at the central endings of these neurons in the spinal cord activates pain pathways.

    b. Release at the peripheral endings results in 'neurogenic inflammation' [see ✎ p. 200].

13. Opioid peptides, angiotensin II, oxytocin, bradykinin, vasopressin, gonadotrophin-releasing hormone, substance P, VIP, cholecystokinin, bombesin [see ✎ Table 9.1].

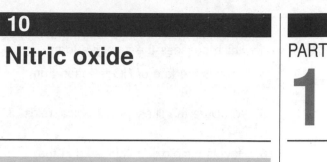

10
Nitric oxide

PART 1

BACKGROUND INFORMATION

Nitric oxide, NO, is an important signalling molecule and its release from the endothelium, in response to agonist action or shear stress, or from NANC nerves, in response to action potentials, mediates relaxation of vascular or visceral smooth muscle. Activation of guanylate cyclase, leading to an increase in the intracellular concentration of cGMP underlies this action. The cytotoxic actions of NO result from its conversion to the reactive species 'peroxynitrite' which can destroy invading organisms.

NO is a diffusible gas and is not stored in the tissues; rather it is produced on demand by **nitric oxide synthase**. Constitutive and inducible forms of this enzyme are found. The activity of the constitutively active enzyme is enhanced by a rise in $[Ca^{2+}]_i$ and this can explain the release of NO from the endothelium by Ca^{2+}-mobilising agonists and from nerve endings by action potentials. NO is produced from endogenous arginine, and arginine analogues (e.g. L-NMMA) can inhibit its production. The pharmacological importance of NO relates to its release by 'nitric oxide donors' such as glyceryl trinitrate and nitroprusside, which have valuable vasodilator actions. In addition, nitric oxide synthase inhibitors and inhaled NO have potential therapeutic value.

QUESTIONS

1. Name three agonists which can produce vasodilatation, at least in part, by stimulating the release of NO from the vascular endothelium.

2. What are the differences between the constitutive and inducible forms of nitric oxide synthase?

3. Name three tissues which possess the constitutive form of the enzyme and three which possess the inducible form.

4. What is the fate of NO released from cells?

5. What are the likely physiological roles of NO?

6. How is nitric oxide implicated in the excitotoxicity of glutamate?

7. What are the potential uses of NO and NO donors?

8. Which of the following statements are true and which false?

   A. The synthesis of NO can be inhibited by L-N-monomethyl arginine.

   B. Nitric oxide has a very short plasma half-life (5–10 min).

   C. Nitric oxide synthase inhibitors have valuable antihypertensive actions.

   D. Nitric oxide promotes platelet aggregation.

   E. The inducible form of nitric oxide synthase is calcium-dependent.

   F. Superoxide dismutase will reduce the toxic effects of NO.

   G. NO elevates the tissue concentration of cGMP by inhibiting the phosphodiesterase.

ANSWERS

1. **Bradykinin**, **ACh**, **substance P**, **adenosine diphosphate**.

2. The constitutive enzyme, unlike the inducible, is Ca^{2+}-dependent. The inducible enzyme produces more NO than the constitutive form. Glucocorticoids inhibit formation of the inducible form but have no effect on the constitutive form [see 📖 Table 10.1].

3. The constitutive enzyme is found in endothelial cells, platelets, osteoblasts, peripheral (NANC) and some CNS neurons. The inducible enzyme is found in macrophages, neutrophils, fibroblasts, vascular smooth muscle and endothelial cells [see 📖 pp. 205–206].

4. Most NO is rapidly oxidised to nitrate via nitrite, some will bind to macromolecules, e.g. haemoglobin, and a proportion is converted to more stable nitrosothiols [see 📖 p. 206].

5. NO release from the endothelium will influence regional blood flow and may have a more general role in the control of blood pressure. In the nervous system NO may serve as a transmitter or neuromodulator. NO, released from white blood cells, is converted to reactive products which kill invading microorganisms. [see 📖 Table 10.2, p. 209 box]

6. Glutamate excitotoxicity is thought to be mediated by an elevation of $[Ca^{2+}]_i$ caused by Ca^{2+} entry through NMDA receptor channels. The activation of constitutive NOS by Ca^{2+} generates NO which under suitable redox conditions is converted to peroxynitrite which produces lethal cell damage [see 📖 Fig. 10.3].

7. NO donors (e.g. **nitroprusside**, **glyceryl trinitrate**) are well-established therapeutic agents with important actions in angina and hypertension. Inhaled NO may be of benefit in adult respiratory distress syndrome [see 📖 p. 209].

8. **A**. True; L-NMMA is a competitive substrate [see 📖 p. 210].

   B. True; it is taken up avidly by haemoglobin and is also rapidly converted to nitrite and nitrate [see 📖 pp. 206, 210].

   C. False; NOS inhibitors would have the opposite effect, blocking any existing NO-mediated vasorelaxation [see 📖 pp. 208, 209 box].

   D. False; nitric oxide *inhibits* platelet aggregation [see 📖 p. 209 box].

E. False; it is the constitutively active form which is activated by Ca²⁺-calmodulin [see 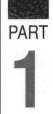 Fig. 10.2].

F. True; superoxide dismutase reduces the concentration of superoxide anion which is required for the production of the toxic peroxynitrite [see Fig. 10.3].

G. False; NO activates guanylate cyclase [see p. 206].

Local hormones, inflammation and allergy

BACKGROUND INFORMATION

The term 'inflammatory reaction' refers to the local events which occur in response to a disease-causing organism (pathogen). It consists of immunologically specific reactions superimposed on innate (non-immunological) reactions. These reactions have survival value but if inappropriately deployed they are deleterious.

Many of the conditions which a doctor is called on to treat are the result of such inappropriately deployed inflammatory/immune responses. It is therefore important to understand the mediators which control these responses since drugs currently used (and many drugs in the pipeline) are directed at influencing the generation and/or action of these mediators.

The inflammatory reaction involves both vascular and cellular events. Mediators are derived from both plasma and cells, and in turn modify both vascular and cellular events. The cells are white blood cells (e.g. neutrophils, lymphocytes, monocytes) and tissue cells (e.g. mast cells, macrophages). The mediators derived from cells include **eicosanoids**, **platelet-activating factor**, **cytokines**, **histamine**, **neuropeptides**, and many others; those derived from plasma include **complement components** and components of the **kinin** cascade.

The specific immunological response (for which the key cells are lymphocytes) has an induction phase and an effector phase. The effector phase consists of an antibody-mediated component and a cell-mediated component. During the induction phase, B cells, which recognise a foreign antigen (such as a bacterial product) respond by proliferating and then synthesising specific antibodies that can interact with the antigen; T cells respond by giving rise to cytotoxic T cells (which kill virus-containing host cells) and Tlk cells which produce lympho-

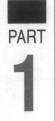

PART

1

kines such as γ-interferon (which enables macrophages to kill organisms like the tubercle bacillus). Allergy or hypersensitivity reactions result when the immune response is inappropriately triggered. Four types of hypersensitivity reactions are recognised, three being due to inappropriate antibody-mediated reactions and one being due to inappropriate cell-mediated reactions.

A summary chart of the mediators derived from phospholipids, with their principal actions, the main drugs which inhibit their generation and examples of analogues of the mediators which are used as drugs, is given in Chapter 12 (Fig. 9)

QUESTIONS

1. Two important inflammatory mediators are derived by the following mechanisms:

   a. .... by enzyme action on a plasma component ....;

   b. .... released preformed from .... cells by .... or ....

2. Define the terms 'eicosanoid' and 'prostanoid'.

3. **a.** What inflammatory mediators are generated by enzyme action on membrane phospholipids?

   b. What are the pathways involved?

   c. What are the main sites at which currently used drugs influence the generation or action of these mediators?

4. What are the main pharmacological actions of histamine? What are the main pathophysiological roles of histamine for which treatment is indicated? What receptors are involved in each role?

5. Which inflammatory mediator causes vasodilatation, increases vascular permeability, is a chemotaxin for white blood cells, activates and aggregates platelets and is a spasmogen on most smooth muscle?

6. How are the prostanoid receptors classified?

7. Which **prostanoids** are involved mainly in vascular responses and haemostatic mechanisms and what are their actions?

8. What are the main pharmacological actions of **PGE$_2$**?

9. What are the main pathophysiological roles of the **leukotrienes**?

10. How is the action of:

    a. bradykinin, b. histamine, c. PGI$_2$ terminated?

11. What are the main actions of **bradykinin**?

12. Define cytokine.

13. What cytokine is particularly important in the inflammatory reaction in a rheumatoid joint?

14. Which inflammatory mediator is a nonapeptide? Which inflammatory mediator is stored preformed?

15. Which of the following statements are true, and which false? If you think a statement is false, explain why.

    A. Histamine causes increased vascular permeability by an action on the capillaries.

    B. Preformed **PGE$_2$** is a mediator released during the acute inflammatory reaction.

    C. LTD$_4$ is derived enzymically from **LTC$_4$**.

    D. LTC$_4$ is derived enzymically from **LTB$_4$**.

    E. The **elcosanoids** and **PAF** are derived from arachidonate.

    F. Angiotensin-converting enzyme:

    (i) inactivates a vasodilator and (ii) activates a vasoconstrictor.

    G. Some of the actions of **bradykinin** are due to released **prostaglandin E$_2$**.

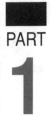

H. Some of the actions of **prostaglandin E$_2$** are due to the release of mast cell **histamine**.

I. Some of the results of activation of mast cells by antigen reacting with cell-fixed antibody are due to **prostaglandin D$_2$** release.

J. Complement component, **C5a**, causes mast cell **histamine** release by action on specific complement receptors.

K. Morphine causes mast cell histamine release by an action on specific morphine receptors.

L. PGI$_2$ causes vasodilatation and increased vascular permeability.

M. PGF$_{2\alpha}$ causes contraction of uterine muscle.

N. PGD$_2$ acts as a spasmogen in the bronchi by direct stimulant action of **PGD$_2$** receptors on smooth muscle.

O. PGD$_2$ aggregates platelets.

ANSWERS

1. a. Bradykinin is generated by kallikrein action on a plasma kininogen (which is an α-globulin) [see 🖉 p. 241 box].

b. Histamine is released from mast cells by complement components **C3a** or **C5a** or by reaction of antigen with cell-fixed IgE antibody [see 🖉 p. 229 box].

2. Eicosanoids are mediators derived from 20-carbon essential fatty acids, the most abundant in man being 5,8,11,14-eicosatetraenoic acid, arachidonic acid. The term prostanoid refers, strictly speaking, only to the prostaglandins but is often used to encompass both prostaglandins and thromboxanes [see 🖉 p. 231].

3. a. The **eicosanoids** and **PAF**.

b, c. Cyclo-oxygenase can be inhibited by **non-steroidal anti-inflammatory drugs**. **Glucocorticoids** inhibit

phospholipase A$_2$ (and therefore both arachidonate and PAF generation) by directing synthesis of a PLA$_2$ inhibitor, lipocortin 1 and possibly by other as yet unknown mechanisms [see 🖉 p. 232 box, Figs 11.5, 11.7, 11.8, 11.9].

4. Histamine stimulates gastric acid secretion (H$_2$), contracts most smooth muscle (H$_1$), causes vasodilatation (H$_1$, H$_2$), increases vascular permeability (H$_1$), stimulates the heart (H$_2$) [see 🖉 p. 229 box].

The main pathophysiological role of **histamine** is as a stimulant of gastric acid secretion, which causes pain and damage in peptic ulcer. Treatment is by H$_2$-receptor antagonists, e.g. **cimetidine** [see 🖉 Figs 19.2, 19.3, 19.5]. Histamine is also the main mediator in type 1 hypersensitivity reactions, e.g. urticaria, hay fever; treatment is by H$_1$-receptor antagonists [see 🖉 p. 229 box, Table 12.4].

5. PAF [see 🖉 p. 238 box, Fig. 11.5].

6. There are five main prostanoid receptors, one each for the five natural prostanoids: **PGE$_2$**, **PGI$_2$**, **PGD$_2$**, **PGF$_{2\alpha}$**, **TXA$_2$**—termed EP, IP, DP, FP, TP receptors respectively. There are three subgroups of EP receptor, EP$_1$, EP$_2$, EP$_3$ [see 🖉 p. 233].

7. PGI$_2$ and **TXA$_2$** are a Ying-Yang pair of particular importance in haemostasis and thrombosis. PGI$_2$ is generated by vascular endothelium and causes vasodilatation and inhibition of platelet adhesion and aggregation; TXA$_2$ is released from platelets and causes platelet aggregation and vasoconstriction. TXA$_2$ is important in blood clotting (and also thrombosis). PGI$_2$ stops platelets sticking to normal vascular endothelium [see 🖉 p. 234 box].

8. Inhibition of gastric acid secretion, vasodilatation, inhibition of activation of inflammatory cells, stimulation of uterine muscle [see 🖉 p. 234 box].

9. LTB$_4$ is a potent chemotaxin and activator of white blood cells in areas of

inflammation. The cysteinyl-leukotrienes (**LTC$_4$**, **LTD$_4$**, **LTE$_4$**) cause contraction of bronchial smooth muscle, vasoconstriction of coronary vessels; they are held to be important in asthma and possibly coronary insufficiency [see 📓 p. 237 box].

10. **a. Bradykinin** is inactivated mainly by the angiotensin-converting enzyme (kininase II) in the lung, also by kininase I in serum [see 📓 p. 239].

   b. Histamine is inactivated by local histaminase and/or imidazole N-methyltransferase [see 📓 p. 227].

   c. PGI$_2$ is inactivated by hydrolysis in the lung [see 📓 p. 233].

11. Vasodilatation (partly through generation of PGs), increased vascular permeability, contraction of most smooth muscle, stimulation of pain nerve endings [see 📓 p. 241 box].

12. **Cytokines** are peptide regulators of inflammatory and immune responses released from activated inflammatory and immune cells and acting on other inflammatory/immune cells. They constitute intercellular messengers which influence the immune system and integrate its function with other physiological systems [see 📓 p. 244 box].

13. **IL-1** is particularly important as a mediator in rheumatoid joint inflammation [see 📓 p. 243].

14. **Bradykinin** is a nonapeptide [see 📓 p. 239]. **Histamine** is stored preformed [see 📓 p. 227].

15. **A.** False; **histamine** causes increased permeability by an action on the postcapillary venules *not* the capillaries [see 📓 p. 229].

   B. False; **PGE$_2$** is not stored preformed, it is synthesised when cells are damaged.

   C. True [see 📓 Fig. 11.5].

   D. False; from **LTA$_4$** [see 📓 Fig. 11.5].

E. False; eicosanoids are derived from arachidonate and both arachidonate and **PAF** are derived from phospholipid [see 📓 Figs 11.5, 11.7].

F. True; it inactivates **bradykinin** and it generates **angiotensin II** from angiotensin I [see 📓 p. 239].

G. True; it can activate phospholipase A$_2$ [see Answer 11 above].

H. False; **PGE$_2$** actually inhibits release of mast cell histamine, by increasing intracellular cyclic AMP in the mast cell.

I. True [see 📓 p. 234].

J. True [see 📓 p. 227].

K. False; **morphine** can cause histamine release, by virtue of being a base, not because it acts on morphine receptors [see 📓 p. 227].

L. False; **PGI$_2$** is a potent vasodilator, but does not itself directly increase vascular permeability; its action as a vasodilator potentiates the effect of **bradykinin** and **histamine** which do increase vascular permeability [see 📓 p. 234].

M. True; it is implicated in spasmodic dysmenorrhoea [see 📓 p. 233 and Ch. 22].

N. False; **PGD$_2$** relaxes vascular, uterine and gastrointestinal tract muscle by a direct action on DP receptors, but causes bronchoconstriction by an action on thromboxane receptors. [Note that there is only a summarised version of this in 📓 Fig. 11.5 and p. 234 box; full details are given in the text.]

O. False; **PGD$_2$** inhibits platelet aggregation [see 📓 p. 233].

12

Drugs used to suppress inflammatory and immune reactions

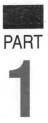

BACKGROUND INFORMATION

Inflammatory and immune reactions are essentially basic biological mechanisms for dealing with invading pathogens, but these reactions may themselves cause damage if they are inappropriately activated. Many diseases are the result of these inappropriately activated inflammatory and immune responses. The drugs used to deal with these conditions are the glucocorticoids [see p. 72], the non-steroidal anti-inflammatory drugs (NSAIDs), the disease-modifying antirheumatoid drugs (DMARDs), drugs used to treat gout, the immunosuppressants and histamine H_1-receptor antagonists.

NSAIDs (e.g. **ibuprofen, naproxen, piroxicam**), in addition to having greater or lesser degrees of anti-inflammatory action, are also able to lower a raised body temperature (i.e. are antipyretic) and can reduce some types of pain (i.e. are mildly analgesic). Furthermore, one NSAID, **aspirin**, also has significant effects on blood clotting and is important in the treatment (and in some cases the prevention) of thromboembolic disease [see p. 175].

DMARDs (e.g. **penicillinamine, gold compounds, chloroquine**) and the **glucocorticoids** can relieve symptoms and can slow the progress of rheumatoid disease but do not cure it.

The drugs used to treat gout act by inhibiting leucocyte migration into joints (**colchicine**) and/or by general anti-inflammatory actions (**NSAIDs**), and/or by inhibiting either the synthesis of uric acid (**allopurinol**) or its excretion (**probenecid**).

Histamine H_1-receptor antagonists (e.g. **terfenadine**): histamine has pro-inflammatory effects by action mainly on H_1-receptors on blood vessels and smooth muscle. In view of the central place accorded to histamine in inflammatory reactions by many pathologists, you may well find it surprising that current H_1-receptor antagonists have no significant anti-inflammatory actions. They are, however, reasonably effective in type I hypersensitivity reactions (hay fever, urticaria). A CNS action that is often termed a side effect, sedation (occurring with some H_1-antagonists e.g. **promethazine**), can be therapeutically useful, as can a central anti-emetic action such as occurs, e.g. with **diphenydramine**, which is made use of in the treatment of motion sickness.

Immunosuppressant drugs include **glucocorticoids, cyclosporin, azathiaprine** and **cyclophosphamide** [see ✒ Chs 21, 36].

Figure 9 gives a summary chart of phospholipid-derived mediators, specifying their principal actions, examples of the main drugs which inhibit their synthesis and clinically useful prostanoid analogues.

QUESTIONS

1. What is the primary mechanism of action of the **NSAIDs**?

2. How is the primary mechanism of action of the **NSAIDs** related to:

   a. their anti-inflammatory action; **b.** their analgesic effects; **c.** their antipyretic effect?

3. What are the main therapeutic indications for **NSAIDs**?

4. In what patients should **NSAIDs** either not be given or be used only with care?

5. What are the common general unwanted actions of **NSAIDs**?

6. The **NSAID a.** .... can precipitate an encephalitis in children with viral infections. The **NSAID b.** .... has only weak anti-inflammatory actions but is an effective analgesic in pains associated with vascular changes (e.g. headache).

7. Give four examples of important and/or commonly used **NSAIDs** other than aspirin, giving an indication of the anti-inflammatory potency.

41

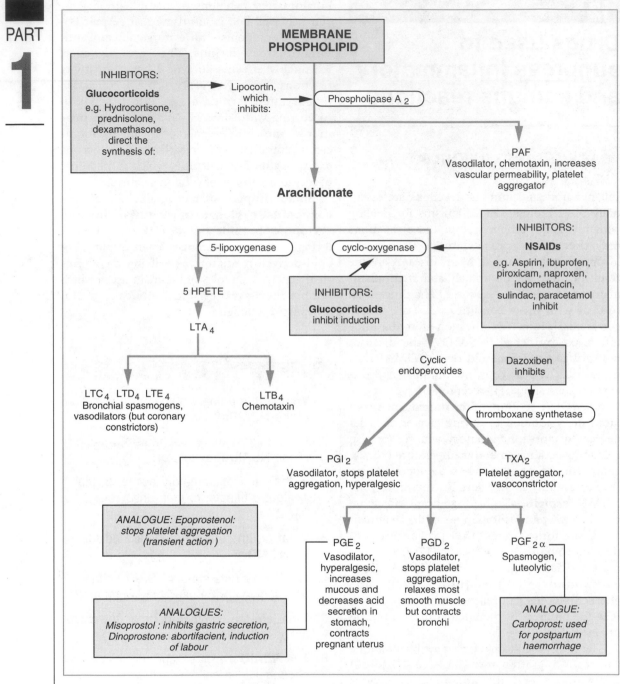

Fig. 9 Summary chart of the mediators derived from membrane phospholipids with their principal actions, the main drugs which inhibit their generation and analogues of the mediators which are used as drugs.

8. Give examples of **H$_1$-receptor antagonists** which have: **a.** considerable sedative action; **b.** selective H$_1$-receptor antagonism, with no effects on muscarinic receptors.

9. How does **cyclosporin** work?

10. Indicate which of the following statements are true and which false. If you think a statement is false, explain why.

A. The anti-inflammatory action of **NSAIDs** is due to direct inhibition of accumulation of inflammatory cells.

B. The main mechanism of action of **NSAIDs** is inhibition of cyclo-oxygenase.

C. Paracetamol is a first-line agent for treatment of an acutely inflamed joint.

D. Naproxen is reported to precipitate an encephalitis in children with viral infections.

E. Piroxicam has a long half-life.

F. Benorylate is an aspirin–paracetamol ester broken down into these constituents in the gastrointestinal tract.

G. NSAIDs are very likely to cause gastrointestinal disturbances because they abrogate the protective effect of PGE$_2$ on gastric mucosa.

H. Large doses of **salicylates** can upset the body's acid–base balance.

I. NSAIDs have analgesic action because, by decreasing PAF generation, they decrease PAF-mediated sensitisation of nociceptive nerve endings to **bradykinin** and **5-HT**.

J. Colchicine is effective in acute rheumatic joint disease.

K. The main effect of overdosage with **paracetamol** is bone marrow depression.

L. Combined therapy with gold preparations and penicillamine is advantageous in rheumatoid disease since their actions are synergistic.

M. Acute exacerbations of rheumatoid arthritis necessitate treatment with either **penicillamine** or **gold** in order to produce immediate benefit.

N. Allopurinol increases uric acid excretion.

O. NSAIDs such as **indomethacin** are effective in acute attacks of gout, but aspirin is contraindicated.

P. Colchicine acts by increasing uric acid secretion in the proximal tubule.

Q. Diphenhydramine is a specific antagonist on H$_1$-receptors.

R. Astemizole is a long-acting H$_1$-antagonist.

S. Terfenadine is an H$_1$-receptor antagonist with virtually no sedative action.

T. The H$_1$-antagonist, **cyclizine**, can be used for motion sickness.

U. The peripheral muscarinic antagonist actions of some H$_1$-antagonists are sometimes clinically useful.

V. H$_1$-antagonists are drugs of choice in relaxing asthmatic bronchospasm.

W. A good drug for treating hay fever is **promethazine** since (i) it has no sedative action and (ii) it is long-acting.

X. The immunosuppressive effect of **cyclosporin** is mainly due to its effects on T lymphocytes.

Y. Cyclosporin has to be given by i.v. infusion.

Z. NSAIDs inhibit 5-lipoxygenase, and thus reduce leukotriene synthesis.

ANSWERS

1. Any tissue/cell damage, such as occurs in an area of inflammation, results in profuse generation of prostanoids which flood out into the surrounding tissue. All **NSAIDs** act by inhibiting cyclo-

PART

1

43

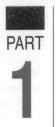

PART

1

oxygenase (COX) which acts on arachidonate to produce cyclic endoperoxides which in turn give rise to the prostanoids. There are two COX enzymes, viz. COX-1 and COX-2, the first being constitutively expressed in most tissues, the latter being induced in activated inflammatory. cells. Currently available NSAIDs act on both COX-1 and COX-2. They decrease the production of all the prostanoids, which are mediators that not only have potent pro-inflammatory effects in their own right but also potentiate the action of other inflammatory mediators such as **histamine** and **bradykinin** [see ✐ Ch. 11, Figs 11.5, 11.8].

2. **a.** The *anti-inflammatory action* of NSAIDs (probably brought about mainly by inhibition of COX-2) is due mainly to the decrease in the production of the vasodilator PGs, viz. **PGE$_2$**, **PGI$_2$**, which results in less vasodilatation and, indirectly, less oedema; less potentiation of the actions of histamine and bradykinin is also a factor.

   b. The *analgesic* effect occurs because the reduced PG generation means less sensitisation of nociceptive nerve endings to **bradykinin**, **5-hydroxy-tryptamine**, etc. [see ✐ pp. 248, 617 box, Ch. 31, Fig. 31.5].

   c. The *antipyretic* effect is related to the decrease, in the hypothalamus, of **PGE$_2$**—the mediator which raises the set-point of temperature control in fever [see ✐ p. 248].

3. The main therapeutic indications of the NSAIDs:

   a. Aspirin is important in the treatment, and prevention of recurrence, of coronary thrombosis [see ✐ pp. 254 box, 344, 348 box].

   b. Most **NSAIDs** can be used, long term, for relief of the symptoms of inflammation (pain, swelling) in a wide variety of musculoskeletal and joint diseases (e.g. rheumatoid arthritis) [see ✐ p. 255 box].

   c. Most **NSAIDs** can be used, short term, for the relief of mild to moderate pain (e.g. headache, dysmenorrhoea), especially if there has been some tissue damage (e.g. post-operation pain). **Indomethacin** should not be used for mild conditions [see Answer 7, below].

4. **NSAIDs** should not be given to patients with active peptic ulcers; they must be used with care in the elderly and avoided if possible in patients with asthma.

5. The general unwanted effects of **NSAIDs** (seen particularly if used long term) are gastrointestinal disturbances (common), and hypersensitivity reactions (e.g. skin rashes). Liver disorders, bone marrow depression and renal damage are less common. It is now thought that these unwanted effects are due to inhibition of COX-1 [see ✐ p. 252 box].

6. **a. Aspirin** can precipitate an encephalitis in children with viral infections [see ✐ p. 247, Table 12.1].

   b. Paracetamol has weak anti-inflammatory actions but is useful for headache [see ✐ p. 250].

7. Commonly used NSAIDs include: **piroxicam** (potent anti-inflammatory action), **ibuprofen**, **naproxen** (moderate potency). **Indomethacin** is very potent and is less commonly used [see ✐ Tables 12.1, 12.3].

8. **a. Diphenhydramine** and **promethazine** are H$_1$-receptor antagonists with marked sedative action.

   b. Terfenadine is selective for the H$_1$-receptor [see ✐ Table 12.4].

9. **Cyclosporin** inhibits T helper cell function in the induction phase of the immune response [see ✐ p. 262, Figs 11.3, 11.4].

10. **A.** False; they have little if any direct effect [see ✐ p. 251 box—but see Answer Z below].

    B. True.

C. False; **paracetamol** is not anti-inflammatory and will have little effect in the presence of large numbers of leucocytes [see 🔖 p. 255 box].

D. False; **aspirin** may do this [see 🔖 Table 12.1].

E. True; $t_{1/2}$ is about 45 hours.

F. False; it is broken down in the liver. [There is a misprint in 🔖 Table 12.1 but this is stated correctly in the text on 🔖 p. 255].

G. True [see 🔖 p. 252 box].

H. True [see 🔖 p. 253].

I. False; this statement would be true if PGE_2 were substituted for PAF.

J. False; **colchicine** is used in gout [see 🔖 p. 258].

K. False; overdosage of **paracetamol** causes serious liver damage [see 🔖 p. 255 box].

L. False; **penicillamine** is a metal chelator and will reduce the effect of gold preparations [see 🔖 p. 256].

M. False; with both agents, action develops slowly over several months [see 🔖 pp. 256, 257].

N. False; **allopurinol** inhibits uric acid synthesis by inhibiting xanthine oxidase [see 🔖 p. 258].

O. True; **aspirin** antagonises uricosuric drugs [see 🔖 p. 254].

P. False; it decreases leucocyte migration into the gouty joint [see 🔖 p. 259].

Q. False; it also has marked muscarinic-receptor antagonism [see 🔖 Table 12.4].

R. True [see 🔖 Table 12.4].

S. True [see 🔖 Table 12.4].

T. True [see 🔖 pp. 261, 395].

U. False; the *central* antimuscarinic effects may be useful, e.g. in motion

sickness, but who wants blurred vision, constipation, retention of urine and a dry mouth?

V. False; some new H_1-antagonists may be useful adjuncts to other anti-asthma drugs [see 🔖 p. 363].

W. False; this would be true for **astemizole** [see 🔖 Table 12.3].

X. True; [see 🔖 p. 262].

Y. False; it can also be given orally [see 🔖 p. 262].

Z. False. (According to some recent experimental work, two NSAIDs, **indomethacin** and **diclofenac**, can reduce leukotriene generation indirectly, by promoting arachidonate reincorporation into triglycerides in leucoctyes and synovial cells; but this is small print stuff.)

PART

1

45

13

The heart

BACKGROUND INFORMATION

The main clinical disorders of the heart include cardiac failure, dysrhythmias and angina pectoris. Understanding of the causes of these disorders requires prior understanding of the cardiac muscle action potential, myocardial contraction, coronary flow and autonomic control of the heart. Calcium is intimately involved in many of these processes.

Drugs used clinically include:

For cardiac failure: the cardiac glycosides, digoxin and digitoxin. The main result of the action of these agents is increased calcium concentration inside the cells, thereby increasing contraction and cardiac output. (ACE inhibitors and diuretics are also used in this condition; considered further in Chs 14 and 18.)

For angina: organic nitrates (e.g. **glyceryl trinitrate**) relax smooth muscle causing vasodilatation; β-adrenoceptor antagonists (e.g. **atenolol**) and calcium antagonists (e.g. **diltiazem**) reduce oxygen consumption and the latter also cause coronary vasodilatation.

For dysrhythmias: there are four classes of antidysrhythmic drugs:

I. Na^+-channel blockers such as **quinidine** and **lignocaine**
II. β-receptor antagonists such as **propranolol** and **atenolol**
III. Agents which prolong the myocardial refractory period such as **amiodarone**
IV. Calcium antagonists such as **verapamil** and **diltiazem**.

QUESTIONS

1. a. What is the basic physiopathological basis of re-entry dysrhythmias?

b. What are the main factors favouring the production of abnormal pacemaker activity?

c. What is heart block?

2. Give an example of a drug that enhances cardiac contractility by an action on Na^+-ion movement.

3. About what percentage of cardiac output is used to perfuse the heart itself through the coronary circulation?

4. a. What is angina pectoris?

b. What mediators are thought to be responsible for anginal pain?

5. How might drug treatment prevent damage after coronary occlusion?

6. What is atrial natriuretic peptide and what is its principal action?

7. What are the effects of sympathetic stimulation on the heart? What receptor is involved?

8. What are the effects of parasympathetic stimulation on the heart? What receptor is involved?

9. Name the main cardiac glycosides.

10. a. List the four main cardiac actions of cardiac glycosides. Which is an unwanted effect?

b. List the main unwanted non-cardiac effects of the cardiac glycosides.

11. What is the mechanism of action of the cardiac glycosides on the heart muscle?

12. a. What are the differences between the individual cardiac glycosides?

b. Which is most commonly used clinically?

c. What are the main therapeutic uses?

13. What is the mode of action of amrinone and milrinone?

14. With respect to antidysrhythmic drugs, what is use-dependence?

15. Class I antidysrhythmic drugs are subdivided into three subclasses. Give examples of drugs in each subclass, specifying how they differ.

16. What is the rationale for the use of β_1-antagonists in the treatment of dysrhythmias?

17. **a.** Give an example of a class III antidysrhythmic drug. How does it differ from other antidysrhythmic agents in terms of onset of action?

    b. Give two examples of class IV drugs. How do they work?

18. There are three classes of drug used in angina. What are they and what is the main action of each class?

19. **a.** Name two important organic nitrates used in treating heart disease.

    b. What is the mechanism of the vasodilator action of the nitrates?

    c. What side effects may occur with large doses of the nitrates?

    d. What is the basis of their effectiveness in relieving angina?

20. Name two calcium antagonists used in treating heart disease.

21. The major effects of calcium antagonists are on the heart and vascular smooth muscle. Why don't they block skeletal muscle contraction, neurotransmitter release, hormonal release, etc, since all of these require influx of calcium?

22. There are thought to be two main types of Ca^{2+} channel through which Ca^{2+} enters vascular smooth muscle. What are they and which one is the site of action of Ca^{2+} antagonists?

23. What is the difference in distribution of L-type and N-type calcium channels?

24. What are the main sites of action of **verapamil**, **nifedipine** and **diltiazem**?

25. What are the clinical uses of calcium antagonists? Indicate the basis of their use in each condition specified.

26. The main therapeutic aims in the treatment of angina pectoris are (a) to decrease cardiac work, (b) to increase perfusion of the heart muscle. Outline briefly the extent to which the commonly used anti-anginal drugs fulfil these aims. Which classes of anti-anginal drugs can be usefully combined and which should not be?

ANSWERS

1. **a.** There is continuous circulation of the impulse [see 📖 Fig. 13.3].

    b. (i) The action of catecholamines, which increase excitability of cardiac cells.

    (ii) Ischaemic damage which causes partial depolarisation [see 📖 p. 272].

    c. Partial or complete block of conduction through the AV nodes or bundle of His. Atria and ventricles beat independently [see 📖 p. 273].

2. Cardiac glycosides, via Na^+/K^+ pump inhibition, increase $[Na]_i$ and indirectly increase Ca^{2+} levels [see 📖 p. 274].

3. 4%. Surprisingly, when one takes into account its metabolic needs, the heart is one of the most poorly perfused tissues in the body.

4. **a.** The condition in which the O_2 supply to heart muscle is inadequate for its needs, resulting in characteristic chest pains.

    b. K^+, H^+, prostaglandins, bradykinin, adenosine, ADP, PGs. Note the parallels with cutaneous pain mediation [see 📖 p. 278].

5. Therapeutic approaches which (used with caution) might have this effect include reducing the workload on the heart by the use of a β_1-antagonist or vasodilator, or preventing Ca^{2+} influx by the use of Ca^{2+} antagonists [see 📖 p. 278].

6. Atrial natriuretic peptide (ANP) is a hormone released from the atria of the

47

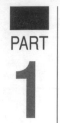

heart in response to volume overload of the circulation. Its main effect is to increase Na^+ excretion by a vasodilator action on the afferent arteriole to the renal glomerulus, increasing filtration pressure [see 🖊 p. 279].

7. • Increased rate (positive chronotropic effect).

 • Increased force of contraction (positive inotropic effect).

 • Increased automaticity.

 • Facilitated AV conduction.

 • Reduced cardiac efficiency.

 The receptor involved is the β_1-adrenoceptor [see Fig. 33, and 🖊 p. 280].

8. • Slowing of the heart.

 • Reduction of automaticity.

 • Reduction of the force of contraction (mainly that of the atria).

 • Inhibition of AV conduction.

 The receptors involved are muscarinic M_2-receptors [see Fig. 33, and 🖊 p. 282].

9. Digoxin, digitoxin and ouabain.

10. **a.** Increased force of contraction

 Block of AV conduction

 Increased vagal activity causing cardiac slowing [see 🖊 p. 285 box]

 Increased ectopic beats; this last is unwanted.

 b. Anorexia, nausea and vomiting, and visual disturbances (yellow-green vision) [see 🖊 p. 285 box].

11. Briefly, they inhibit the Na^+/K^+-ATPase; the $[Na^+]_i$ then rises and Ca^{2+} extrusion is reduced because of a shift in the Na^+/Ca^{2+} exchanger balance. The consequently increased $[Ca^{2+}]_i$ results in greater contraction, so cardiac output increases. (The inhibition of the Na^+/K^+-ATPase also results in a partial depolarisation which has repercussions on cardiac rhythm) [see 🖊 p. 285 box].

12. **a.** **Digoxin** and **digitoxin** each have a long $t_{1/2}$ and are orally effective. **Ouabain**, with a short $t_{1/2}$, is now not used. Digoxin is excreted unchanged, so its effects are influenced by the state of kidney function.

 b. Digoxin is the one most commonly used.

 c. The main therapeutic use is for atrial fibrillation. Another is cardiac failure, though diuretics and vasodilators are of more value for this [see Fig. 33 and 🖊 p. 285 box].

13. Phosphodiesterase inhibition, so increasing cAMP and consequently Ca^{2+} levels. (There is some evidence that these agents may increase mortality) [see Fig. 33 and 🖊 p. 286].

14. This term describes an action of certain class I and class IV drugs which block Na^+ or Ca^{2+} channels; it means that the more often the Na^+ or Ca^{2+} channels are activated, the greater the block, since the drugs bind to the open or refractory state of the channel.

15. Although they all have the same general mechanism of action, namely use-dependent block of Na^+ channels, they are subdivided partly on the basis of their clinical uses as follows:

 Ia for supraventricular tachycardias (e.g. **procainamide**, **quinidine**)

 Ib for ventricular extrasystoles after infarction (e.g. **lignocaine**)

 Ic for ventricular tachycardia (e.g. **flecainide**).

 The functional differences are related to the fact that they dissociate from Na^+ channels at different rates (see 🖊 p. 288].

16. The ventricular dysrhythmias which can occur after myocardial infarction are due in part to a raised sympathetic activity. This increases cardiac excitability by stimulating β_1-adrenoceptors. Beta blockers would reduce this and also tend to slow the heart by reducing the sympathetic effect on the AV node [see 🖊 p. 289].

17. a. Amiodarone. It takes a long time to work [see 🖉 p. 289].

b. Verapamil and **diltiazem** are important examples. They block voltage-gated Ca^{2+} channels and so inhibit the slow inward Ca^{2+} current [see 🖉 p. 289].

18. Organic nitrates—vasodilators

Calcium antagonists—vasodilators

β antagonists—reduce metabolic demand

[see 🖉 p. 292].

19. a. Examples are **glyceryl trinitrate, isosorbide dinitrate, pentaerythritol tetranitrate** (the latter two being longer-acting) [see 🖉 p. 295 box].

b. They relax smooth muscle, especially that of the blood vessels. These drugs are nitric oxide (NO) donors. NO activates guanylate cyclase to increase cGMP which in turn reduces vascular smooth muscle contraction [see 🖉 Fig. 13.15]. Figure 22 shows how cGMP could interfere with a contractile process.

c. Dizziness, throbbing headache and flushing due to relaxation of cutaneous and cerebral vessels [see 🖉 p. 293].

d. (i) They dilate capacitance vessels leading to a reduced pre-load and

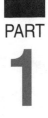

PART

1

DRUGS USED TO TREAT ANGINA PECTORIS:	Decrease cardiac work by:			Increase perfusion of heart muscle
	acting on veins to decrease cardiac filling pressure	acting on arteries to decrease peripheral resistance	decreasing cardiac output	
Nitrates Glyceryl trinitrate, isosorbide dinitrate, pentaerythritol dinitrate	+++	++ Cause fall in blood pressure and thus → Produce tachycardia, (which may be alleviated by beta antagonists)	a secondary fall in cardiac output	+ Dilate collateral vessels
Beta receptor antagonists Propranolol, atenolol, oxprenolol			++ Inhibit NA-mediated inotropic and chronotropic effects	
Calcium channel blockers	Cause decreased calcium influx and thus decreased contraction			
Nifedipine	±	++		
Diltiazem	±	+	±	
Verapamil			+	

Fig. 10 Chart of anti-anginal agents showing the degree to which drugs fulfil the main therapeutic aims for treating angina pectoris, namely decreasing cardiac work or increasing perfusion of the heart muscle. Note that nitrates and beta blockers can be given together but that verapamil and diltiazem can produce excessive bradycardia or heart block if combined with beta antagonists. Dipyridamole may be useful in variant angina.

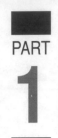
therefore a reduced cardiac output and thus reduced demand for O_2.

(ii) They dilate collateral coronary vessels, which may increase perfusion of ischaemic areas [see 🖉 Fig. 13.16, p. 295 box].

20. **Verapamil**, **nifedipine** and **diltiazem** represent the main agents; there are others [see 🖉 p. 296].

21. There is selectivity for the Ca^{2+} channels (L-type) on cardiovascular tissue, which differ from other types of Ca^{2+} channel [see 🖉 p. 297].

22. Voltage-gated and the putative, receptor-gated channels. The former are the site of action of Ca^{2+} antagonists [see 🖉 p. 296].

23. L-type channels are found mainly in smooth and cardiac muscle and N-type channels mainly in neurons, where they are responsible for the Ca^{2+} influx necessary for neuronal transmitter release. Ca^{2+} antagonists act mainly on L channels. See also Answer 21.

24. **Verapamil** acts mainly on the heart, **nifedipine** on smooth muscle, **diltiazem** on both [see 🖉 p. 297 box].

25. As antidysrhythmic agents: (class IV) **verapamil**, **diltiazem**. Reduction of the transient inward Ca^{2+} current.

    As antihypertensive drugs: **nifedipine**, **diltiazem**. Arteriolar vasodilation and reduced cardiac output.

    As anti-anginal drugs: **diltiazem** and **nifedipine**. Reduction of the cardiac work by lowering peripheral resistance [see 🖉 pp. 297 box, 299 box].

26. See Figure 10.

14
The circulation

BACKGROUND INFORMATION

Numerous endogenous mediators control vascular tone, important agents being noradrenaline, adrenaline, angiotensin II. Others include: dopamine, various prostaglandins, 5-hydroxytryptamine, atrial natriuretic peptide, co-transmitter substances (e.g. VIP, CGRP), endothelin, nitric oxide.

Many pathological conditions involve disturbances in vascular function, examples being hypertension, heart failure, angina pectoris, peripheral vascular disease. A very large number of drugs affect vascular function by a variety of mechanisms. In general there are more agents causing vasodilatation than vasoconstriction and vasodilators are more extensively used clinically.

Drugs can affect vascular smooth muscle in various ways, such as:

By acting directly on the smooth muscle itself:

- on receptors mediating contraction, e.g. α_1-agonists such as **noradrenaline**, α_1-antagonists such as **prazosin**
- on receptors mediating relaxation, e.g. β_2-agonists such as **adrenaline**
- on post-receptor transduction events for contraction, which can be decreased by agents such as **nifedipine** which block the voltage-gated Ca^{2+} channels, and by hyperpolarising agents such as the K^+ channel opener, **diazoxide**
- on post-receptor transduction events for relaxation, which can be increased by nitrates such as **glyceryl trinitrate**.

By acting indirectly on noradrenergic nerve terminals [see Fig. 8 and 🖉 Ch. 7] causing:

- increased NA release, e.g. **amphetamine**
- inhibition of NA re-uptake, e.g. **cocaine**
- decreased NA release, e.g. noradrenergic neuron blockers such as **guanethidine**

- decreased NA synthesis, e.g. α-**methyltyrosine**
- α$_2$-mediated inhibition of NA release, e.g. clonidine (acting mainly in CNS)
- formation of a false transmitter, e.g. α-methylnoradrenaline from **methyldopa** (acting mainly on α$_2$ adrenoceptors in the CNS).

By blocking either the synthesis of angiotensin II, e.g. the angiotensin-converting enzyme inhibitors such as **captopril,** or the action of angiotensin II, e.g. **saralasin**.

By unknown means, e.g. **hydralazine**.

The main internal messenger for contraction is Ca^{2+} and that for relaxation is cyclic AMP. Details of the signal transduction mechanism for contraction and relaxation of smooth muscle are given in Chapter 41 and more details on the vasoactive drugs used to treat hypertension and angina are given in Part 2.

QUESTIONS

1. What are the main uses for vasodilator drugs?

2. What are the main uses for vasoconstrictor drugs?

3. Which vasoactive drugs produce their effects by increasing the concentration of cAMP or cGMP and how do they accomplish this?

4. Which vasoactive drugs produce their effects by direct action on ion channels?

   What are the effects produced and what therapeutic use can be made of them?

5. How are the following drugs given and what are their half-lives:

   hydralazine, diazoxide, nifedipine, sodium nitroprusside, captopril, glyceryl trinitrate?

6. What effects will occur with **dopamine** infusion? What receptors mediate these effects? What clinical use is made of the cardiovascular effects of dopamine?

7. Indicate whether the following statements are true or false. If you think a statement is false, explain why.

A. Saralasin is an angiotensin-converting-enzyme inhibitor.

B. A serious unwanted effect of clinically used Ca^{2+}-channel blockers arises from their effect on neuronal Ca^{2+} channels.

C. Minoxidil is used to treat baldness in men.

D. Cromakalim blocks K^+ channels.

E. Diltiazem blocks all Ca^{2+} channels in both cardiac and smooth muscle.

F. Sodium nitroprusside can give rise to cyanide both in vitro and in vivo.

G. Enalapril increases the concentration of plasma angiotensin I.

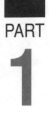

ANSWERS

1. Therapy of hypertension, angina pectoris, cardiac failure and peripheral vascular disease [see 📖 p. 313 box].

2. Used mainly for local effects, e.g. for nasal decongestion, for vasoconstriction with local anaesthetics.

3. Some increase the activity of the adenylate cyclase system by an action on receptors (e.g. β$_2$-**agonists, dopamine**), some by inhibiting the phosphodiesterase which metabolises cAMP (e.g. **xanthines**). **Nitrates** and **sodium nitroprusside** give rise to nitric oxide which activates guanylate cyclase [see 📖 p. 312 box, Fig. 14.1, p. 295 box].

4. Calcium channel blockers block the L-type voltage-dependent calcium channels in vascular smooth muscle, preventing the contractile response to depolarisation. Examples are: **nifedipine, nicardipine** (used in angina and hypertension), **diltiazem** (used in angina), **nimodipine** (used for the cerebral vascular spasm associated with subarachnoid haemorrhage) [see 📖 pp. 312 box, 297 box].

   K^+ channel activators open K^+ channels in the plasma membrane causing

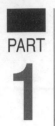

hyperpolarisation and inhibiting action potential generation. Examples are **minoxidil** (used in hypertension), **diazoxide** (used for hypertensive crisis), **cromakalim** and **pinacidil** (still under test) [see 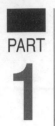 pp. 310–311].

5. **Hydralazine**: orally, $t_{1/2}$ 2–8 h.

   Diazoxide: rapid i.v. injection, $t_{1/2}$ 30 h. (This represents the presence of bound drug; the duration of its antihypertensive action, surprisingly, can be as little as 5 h.)

   Nifedipine: orally, $t_{1/2}$ 2 h.

   Sodium nitroprusside: i.v., $t_{1/2}$ 2 min.

   Captopril: orally, $t_{1/2}$ 1–2 h.

   Glyceryl trinitrate: sublingual tablets or aerosol spray, $t_{1/2}$ 2 h (but effective duration of action 30 min); also given as slow-release tablets for absorption in mouth, by intravenous infusion and by transdermal patch.

   [See 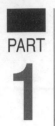 p. 312 box, p. 295.]

6. It acts on β_1-receptors in the heart, α_1-receptors (causing vasoconstriction) in some vessels and dopamine receptors (causing vasodilatation) in renal and mesenteric vessels. It is used to treat cardiogenic shock [see also Fig. 33, and 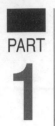 p. 309].

7. **A.** False; it is a competitive antagonist of the vasoconstrictor effects of angiotensin II [see 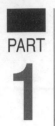 p. 316].

   B. False; the Ca^{2+}-channel blockers used clinically have no obvious effect on neuronal Ca^{2+} channels in vivo. Their main effect is on L channels, which are abundant on smooth muscle and cardiac muscle; they have little or no action on the N channels through which Ca^{2+} enters nerve terminals to trigger transmitter release [see 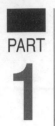 p. 297].

   C. Unlikely as this seems, it is true.

   D. False; it opens them [see 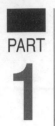 p. 310].

   E. True; the Ca^{2+} channels in both cardiac and smooth muscle are of the L-type, which is sensitive to diltiazem [see 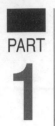 p. 297 box].

   F. True; **sodium nitroprusside** solution can be hydrolysed to cyanide in vitro particularly if exposed to light. In the body, it dissociates into nitric oxide (which is the vasodilator moiety) and cyanide (which is then metabolised to thiocyanate) [see 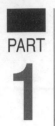 p. 312].

   G. True; it prevents its conversion to **angiotensin II** [see 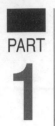 p. 315].

15

Control of lipoprotein metabolism

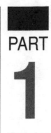

BACKGROUND INFORMATION

Lipids such as cholesterol (C) and triglycerides (T) are transported in the blood complexed with phospholipids, forming lipoproteins. There are four classes of lipoproteins:

- Chylomicrons which transport dietary T and C from the gastrointestinal tract to the tissues (where free fatty acids derived from T are taken up) and thence to the liver, where C is taken up and then stored, oxidised to bile acids, or released into:
- Very Low Density Lipoproteins (VLDL) which transport C and newly synthesised T from liver to tissues where T-derived fatty acids (an important energy source) are taken up, leaving:
- Low Density Lipoproteins (LDL) which now have a large component of C, some of which is taken up by tissues and some by endocytosis of LDL by the liver.
- High Density Lipoproteins absorb C from broken down cells and transfer it to LDL.

Pathological conditions involving increases of plasma lipoproteins are termed hyper-lipidaemias (or hyperlipoproteinaemias). In some types, the cholesterol levels, in particular, are high (hypercholesterolaemia). An increase in plasma cholesterol and its main transporter, LDL, is an important risk factor in athero-sclerosis. One variant of LDL has an apoprotein which decreases fibrinolytic activity and thus could facilitate development of thrombosis.

Drugs can be used to reduce cholesterol and lipoprotein levels, acting as follows:

- by inhibiting cholesterol synthesis (e.g. **simvastatin**)
- by sequestering bile acids in the GIT (e.g. **cholestyramines, colestipol**)

- by altering the relative levels of plasma lipoproteins (e.g. **bezafibrate, gemfibrosil, nicotinic acid**)
- by inhibiting cholesterol absorption from the GIT (e.g. **neomycin**).

QUESTIONS

1. What is the mechanism of action of **cholestyramine**?

2. What is the action of **clofibrate**?

3. What is the mechanism of action of **simvastatin**? How is it administered?

4. Indicate which of the following statements, if any, are true and which false. If you think a statement is false, explain why.

   A. Fibrates act partly by increasing the action of a lipoprotein lipase.

   B. There is still great uncertainty as to whether decreasing LDL-cholesterol will reduce the risk of coronary artery disease.

   C. Nicotinic acid may cause flushing.

   D. Cholestyramine may cause an increased bleeding tendency.

   E. Probucol may cause ventricular tachycardia if used with some antihistamine drugs.

   F. An increased risk of atherosclerosis is associated with hyperlipoproteinaemia.

   G. Some drugs lower the plasma LDL concentration by stimulating synthesis of liver cell LDL receptors and thus increase receptor-mediated endocytosis.

   H. Gemfibrozil can reduce the incidence of coronary heart disease in patients with abnormal concentrations of blood lipids.

   I. Clofibrate is contraindicated in gall bladder disease.

ANSWERS

1. **Cholestyramine** is a resin, a large non-absorbable polymer which binds bile

acids in the gastrointestinal tract and reduces absorption of exogenous cholesterol and increases the metabolism of endogenous cholesterol into bile acids [see 🕮 p. 327, Fig. 15.1].

2. **Clofibrate markedly** decreases VLDL and also produces moderate lowering of LDL and elevation of HDL [see 🕮 Fig. 15.1, p. 327].

3. **Simvastatin** inhibits liver HMG-CoA reductase, the main rate-limiting enzyme in cholesterol synthesis. It is given orally [see 🕮 p. 328, Fig. 15.1].

4. **A.** True [see 🕮 p. 327].

   B. False; there is now fairly good evidence on this point [see 🕮 p. 324].

   C. True [see 🕮 p. 329].

   D. True; with long-continued use it can interfere with the absorption of fat-soluble vitamins and result in a deficiency of vitamin K [see 🕮 p. 327].

   E. True; the drugs in question are astemizole and terfenadine [see 🕮 p. 329].

   F. True [see 🕮 p. 324].

   G. True; this is reported to occur with HMG-CoA reductase inhibitors, as a result of their action in decreasing cholesterol synthesis [see 🕮 p. 328].

   H. True [see p. 327].

   I. True; it can predispose to gallstones [see 🕮 p. 327].

16

Haemostasis and thrombosis

BACKGROUND INFORMATION

Haemostasis is the arrest of blood loss from damaged blood vessels and is crucial for life. Thrombosis is a pathological event. Both involve:
- platelet activity
- blood coagulation (fibrin formation).

Damage or pathology of blood vessels causes loss of endothelium. Platelets then adhere and change shape, flattening and covering the damaged area like sticking plaster. They secrete factors which cause aggregation of more platelets, and negatively charged phospholipids become exposed on the platelet surface. The vascular damage also triggers a complex cascade of coagulation enzymes, the cascade ending in the conversion, by thrombin (factor IIa), of soluble fibrinogen to insoluble fibrin, which forms a mesh that constitutes the framework of the blood clot. The clot is localised to the area of damage because portions of the polypeptide chains of key enzymes are linked by calcium bridges to the negatively charged phospholipids of the adherent platelets. PGI_2 from the surrounding normal endothelium stops platelets adhering and prevents extension of the haemostatic/thrombotic process. A series of inhibitors prevents overshoot of these reactions; a particularly important one is antithrombin III, which neutralises many of the coagulation enzymes. The first enzyme in the coagulation cascade (factor XIIa) also plays a part in starting the clot-dissolving (fibrinolytic) mechanisms.

Drugs can be used to modify haemostasis and thrombosis in three ways:
- by modifying coagulation:
  a. when there is unwanted coagulation; agents which do this are:
     —oral anticoagulants (e.g. **warfarin**)
     —injectable anticoagulants (e.g. **heparin**, and **low-molecular-weight heparins, thrombin inhibitors**)

b. when there are defects in coagulation (e.g. **vitamin K**)

- by modifying platelet aggregation (e.g. **aspirin**)
- by increasing fibrinolysis (e.g. **streptokinase**).

A summary chart of thrombotic mechanisms and the actions of drugs (Fig. 11) is given towards the end of this chapter.

QUESTIONS

1. What are the main events in blood coagulation?

2. Which four coagulation enzymes undergo γ-carboxylation of some of the glutamic acid (Glu) residues at their N terminal ends?

   What is the significance of the γ-carboxylation? What substance, which can be used as a drug, is essential for this process?

3. What is the mechanism of action of **heparin**? Which coagulation enzymes are affected by the action of heparin?

4. How does **warfarin** act? What are the main factors determining the onset of action of warfarin?

5. Will the concentration of prothrombin in the plasma decrease after administration of **warfarin**?

6. What would be the main effect of giving too much **heparin**? What drug could be used to combat this effect and how would it accomplish this?

7. By what mechanisms does **aspirin** modify platelet function?

   Would another NSAID, such as **ibuprofen**, have the same effect?

8. What is the mechanism of action of **streptokinase**?

   What drug could combat the effect of **streptokinase** if too much were given?

   How is streptokinase administered?

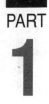

9. The main use of the **a.** .... (state class of antithrombotic drug) is for treating *venous* thromboembolism, using **b.** .... for short-term action, **c.** .... for longer therapy.

   For *arterial* thrombotic disease, such as coronary thrombosis **d.** .... (state class of drug) are used in initial, emergency treatment, given **e.** .... (state route), followed by long-term treatment with **f.** .... (state specific agent), given **g.** .... (state route).

10. What drug can be used (in certain circumstances) for preventing coronary thrombosis, and what are the circumstances?

11. What are the main differences between arterial thrombi and venous thrombi? In what way might these differences influence therapy of arterial and venous thromboembolism?

12. What is **alteplase**? **anistreplase**?

13. Which of the following statements are true and which false?

    (a) Warfarin:

    A. should not be given during the first 3 months of pregnancy.

    B. can be used to prevent clotting of blood collected for laboratory tests on plasma.

    C. is the main anticoagulant used for immediate treatment of myocardial infarction.

    D. has less effect if given with the antibiotic **rifampicin**.

    E. has more effect if given with **oral contraceptives**.

    (b) Streptokinase:

    A. is given by single bolus i.v. injection.

    B. is enzymic, acting as a direct plasminogen activator.

    C. is antigenic.

    D. may cause serious bleeding.

PART 1

E. reduces mortality from myocardial infarction if given soon after onset.

(c) Heparin:

A. is used to prevent deep-vein thrombosis.

B. has immediate onset of action if given i.v.

C. acts by preventing reduction of **vitamin K.**

D. acts by complexing with thrombin and inhibiting it.

ANSWERS

1. See Figure 11.

2. Factors II, VII, IX, X undergo γ-carboxylation, which is essential for interaction of these factors with Ca^{2+} and the negatively charged lipid on the platelet surface; factor V is also necessary. Reduced vitamin K is an essential cofactor in the process [see 📖 p. 335 box, Figs 16.4, 16.5].

3. **Heparin** increases the rate of action of antithrombin III (which inactivates XIIa, XIa, IXa, Xa and IIa) [see 📖 p. 335 box, Fig. 16.2].

4. **Warfarin** prevents reduction of vitamin K and thus inhibits the γ-carboxylation of the glutamic acid residues in factors II, VII, IX, X [see 📖 Fig. 16.5, p. 335]. The onset of action of warfarin depends mainly on the half-lives of the specified factors.

5. The concentration of γ-carboxylated (but not non-γ-carboxylated prothrombin, factor II) would decrease [see 📖 p. 337].

6. Excess **heparin** causes bleeding; it is treated by i.v. protamine sulphate, a basic protein which neutralises heparin [see 📖 p. 341].

7. **Aspirin** acetylates cyclo-oxygenase irreversibly. Platelets cannot synthesise more enzyme and thus their generation of cyclic endoperoxides and of TXA_2 (a potent platelet-aggregating agent) is reduced, whereas vascular endothelium can synthesise more cyclo-oxygenase and therefore generation of PGI_2 (a potent inhibitor of platelet aggregation) recovers. **Ibuprofen** causes reversible inhibition of cyclo-oxygenase and will therefore have only a very transient effect. A summary is given in Figures 9 and 11 [see also 📖 pp. 344 box, 250, Figs 11.5, 11.8].

8. **Streptokinase**, given by i.v. infusion, promotes formation of the fibrinolytic enzyme, plasmin, by forming a complex with plasminogen and gaining enzyme activity. **Tranexamic acid** can inhibit action [see 📖 p. 347, Fig. 16.10, Table 16.1].

9. **a.** anticoagulants, **b.** heparin, **c.** oral anticoagulants/warfarin, **d.** antifibrinolytic drugs, **e.** parenterally, **f.** aspirin, **g.** orally [see 📖 p. 348 box].

10. **Aspirin** can prevent coronary thrombosis where there is known risk of occlusive vascular disease [see 📖 p. 348 box].

11. A venous thrombus is found in slowed/ static blood and consists mainly of blood clot (fibrin meshwork with trapped cells). Arterial thrombi have a 'head' of aggregated platelets (attached to the area of vascular damage) with a tail of blood clot. **Anticoagulants** are used mainly for venous thrombi, **antiplatelet agents** with **fibrinolytic agents** for arterial thrombi [see Answer 9].

12. **Alteplase** is the official name for recombinant tissue-type plasminogen activator (rt-PA); **anistreplase** is the official name for APSAC.

13. (a) **A.** True; it can sometimes be teratogenic [see 📖 p. 339].

    B. False; it only works in vivo [see 📖 p. 337].

    C. False [see Answer 9 above].

    D. True; rifampicin induces the metabolising enzymes [see 📖 Fig. 42.5].

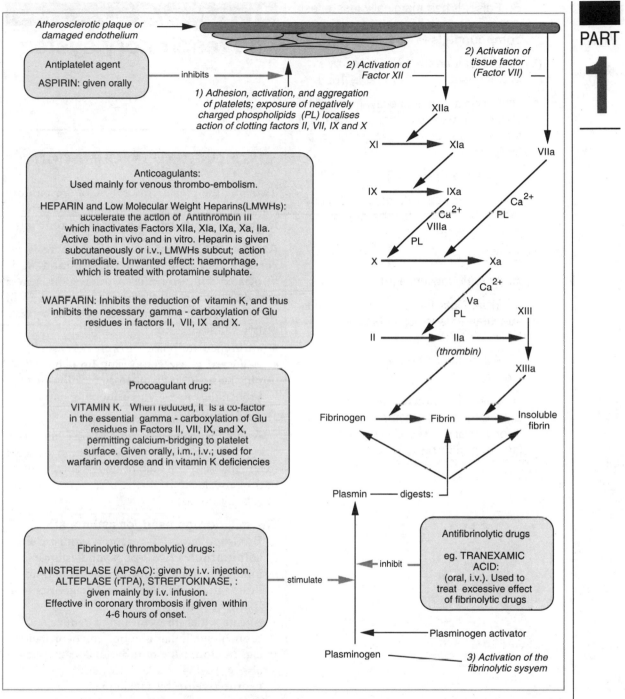

Fig. 11 Summary chart of anticoagulant, antiplatelet, fibrinolytic and antifibrinolytic drugs. A schematic outline of the events (stages 1, 2 and 3) which could occur in an arteriole of the coronary circulation following the development of an atherosclerotic plaque is shown at the top and right-hand side of the diagram and drugs which have an effect on the events depicted are shown in boxes. In treating coronary thrombosis, drugs which increase fibrinolysis are used first, then when the circulation through the affected vessel has been re-established, low-dose aspirin is given daily to prevent recurrence.

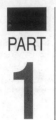

E. False; it has marginally less effect in the presence of **oestrogenic compounds** [see 🖉 p. 339].

(b) A. False; it needs to be given by i.v. infusion [see 🖉 p. 347, Table 16.1].

B. False; it acts indirectly, forming a stable complex with plasminogen and then gains enzymic activity [see 🖉 p. 347].

C. True [see 🖉 p. 347].

D. True; **tranexamic acid** and cross-matched blood should be available [see 🖉 p. 348].

E. True [see 🖉 p. 348].

(c) A. True (in low dosage).

B. True. Note that onset is later after subcutaneous injection [see 🖉 p. 341].

C. False; this is how **warfarin** acts [see 🖉 p. 335 box].

D. False; it increases the action of antithrombin III, a natural inhibitor of thrombin and other clotting factors [see 🖉 p. 335 box].

17

The respiratory system

BACKGROUND INFORMATION

Two of the main disorders of respiratory function are asthma and cough. The latter is frequently associated with chronic bronchitis.

Asthma is a syndrome in which there is reversible recurrent airway obstruction. It is associated with bronchial hyper-responsiveness and there are usually inflammatory changes in the airways. An asthmatic attack often consists of two phases:

- an immediate phase of bronchospasm
- a delayed phase comprising bronchospasm plus an acute inflammatory reaction in the bronchioles in which eosinophils have an important role.

Asthma is increasing in prevalence and has a rising mortality. This may be due to inadequate treatment based on lack of understanding of its pathogenesis; it is not just a type I hyper-sensitivity disease.

The main drugs used for asthma are:

- Bronchodilators: β_2-receptor agonists, e.g. **salbutamol**; cAMP-phosphodiesterase inhibitors, e.g. **theophylline**; second-line drugs: muscarinic-receptor antagonists, e.g **ipratropium**
- Agents which prevent and/or reduce bronchiolar inflammation: glucocorticoids, e.g. **beclomethasone** by inhalation [see also 🖉 p. 434, Table 21.2]; **sodium cromoglycate** by inhalation.

Drugs used for cough include **codeine** and **dextromethorphan**.

QUESTIONS

1. What is the basis of the bronchial hyper-responsiveness in asthmatic subjects?

2. What bronchodilator drugs are used in asthma? Give examples.

3. What intracellular transduction mechanisms are involved in the action of the main bronchodilator drugs?

4. Which anti-asthma drugs can be given by inhalation; which cannot? How are these latter agents given?

5. What non-respiratory actions do the **xanthine drugs** have?

6. Which receptors are involved in the bronchodilator action of **muscarinic-receptor antagonists**?

7. What is the role of **sodium cromoglycate** in the treatment of asthma and what is its mechanism of action?

8. Which anti-asthmatic bronchodilator drugs can be given i.v.; which cannot?

9. What drugs are used to suppress cough?

10. What is **aminophylline**? Does it have any advantages over **theophylline**?

11. Indicate which of the following statements are true, and which false. If you think a statement is false, explain why.

   A. Sodium cromoglycate can be effective treatment of an asthmatic attack.

   B. A common unwanted effect of inhaled **glucocorticoids** is candidiasis (thrush).

   C. β_1-**adrenoceptor agonists** are drugs of first choice for overcoming the bronchospasm of the immediate phase of asthma.

   D. Theophylline relaxes bronchial muscle mainly by antagonism at adenosine receptors.

   E. Dextromethorphan is a cough suppressant particularly useful in treating cough associated with suppurating bronchial inflammation (bronchiectasis).

   F. The preventative action of **sodium cromoglycate** in asthma is due to mast cell stabilisation.

   G. Muscarinic-receptor antagonists are of no use in treating asthma.

   H. Theophylline given by inhalation can be an effective bronchodilator in some cases of asthma.

   I. Salbutamol or **terbutaline**, given by aerosol, are first-line drugs for treatment of the immediate phase of the asthma attack.

   J. Salmeterol is a long-lasting β_2-adrenoceptor agonist causing bronchodilatation lasting up to 12 hours.

   K. Theophylline has a narrow therapeutic 'window', being ineffective below 20 µmol/litre and causing unwanted effects above 110 µmol/litre.

   L. Sustained-release oral **theophylline** preparations can be useful for nocturnal asthma.

   M. FEV_1 is a measure of the fever associated with severe asthma

   N. Acute severe asthma (status asthmaticus) should be treated by rapid i.v. theophylline.

   O. LTD_4 is an important spasmogen in both phases of asthma.

ANSWERS

1. Bronchial hyperresponsiveness is related to the loss of bronchiolar epithelium (caused mainly by eosinophil products) which facilitates local axon reflexes that are triggered by stimulation of irritant receptors to release various peptides; various inflammatory mediators also participate [see ✎ pp. 355–358, Fig. 17.3].

2. Bronchodilators used in asthma: β_2-adrenoceptor agonists (e.g. **salbutamol**, **terbutaline**) and xanthine drugs (e.g. **theophylline**). Muscarinic-receptor antagonists (e.g. **ipratropium**) are adjuncts to other bronchodilators [see ✎ p. 360 box].

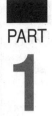

PART

1

3. Both β_2-**receptor agonists** and **xanthine** drugs can cause an increase in intracellular cyclic AMP which activates a protein kinase that has an inhibitory effect on the contractile machinery, thus relaxing spasm. β_2-adrenoceptor agonists increase cAMP by activating adenylate cyclase via a stimulatory G-protein. Xanthine drugs increase cyclic AMP because they inhibit its breakdown by inhibiting cyclic AMP phosphodiesterase: xanthines also increase cyclic GMP [see Ch. 44].

4. Some glucocorticoids (**beclomethasone**) and most β_2-receptor agonists used for bronchodilatation (e.g. **salbutamol**, **terbutaline**) are given by inhalation; as are **sodium cromoglycate** and **ipratropium**. **Xanthine drugs** cannot be so given; they are given orally or by slow i.v. injection [see ✐ p. 360 box, p. 363 box].

5. In addition to bronchodilator actions, **xanthines** act on the CNS to cause increased alertness, stimulate the heart, cause vasodilatation (but some cause cerebral vasoconstriction) and are weak diuretics [see ✐ pp. 359–361].

6. Muscarinic-receptor antagonists (e.g. **ipratropium**) are bronchodilators by virtue of antagonising acetylcholine action on M_3-receptors on smooth muscle, acting mainly in the larger airways [see ✐ p. 353]. But their action is complex. They do not act by decreasing cyclic GMP (as suggested in some books); this would have the opposite effect.

7. **Sodium cromoglycate**, used prophylactically, can prevent both immediate and delayed phases of asthma. It is used particularly in children. It may act by depressing neuronal reflexes [see Answer 2 above], and/or inhibiting **PAF** interaction with platelets and eosinophils. Its effectiveness is probably not due to its ability to inhibit mast cell mediator release [see ✐ p. 363 box, Fig. 17.3].

8. Some β_2-agonists (e.g. **salbutamol**, **terbutaline**) can be given by slow i.v. infusion; most others cannot. Some xanthine drugs, e.g. **theophylline**, are given by slow i.v. infusion; **enprofylline** is given orally. **Ipratropium bromide** is not given i.v. [see ✐ p. 360 box].

9. **Codeine**, **dextromethorphan** [see ✐ p. 364 box].

10. **Aminophylline** is **theophylline ethylenediamine**; it is considerably more soluble than theophylline, and is therefore useful for i.v. injection [see ✐ pp. 359–361].

11. **A.** False; **cromoglycate** is only useful for prevention [see Answer 7 above].

    B. True [see ✐ p. 363 box].

    C. False; β_2-**adrenoceptor agonists** are used. But note that recent guidelines indicate that if a patient finds it necessary to use inhaled β_2-agonists regularly more than once a day, this implies the need for treatment with anti-inflammatory drugs.

    D. False; **theophylline** is an adenosine antagonist but this is not its main mechanism of action in relaxing bronchial muscle [see ✐ p. 360].

    E. False; **dextromethorphan** is a cough suppressant but such agents can cause harmful sputum retention in bronchiectasis.

    F. False; the mechanism of action is not clearly known, but what *is* known is that many compounds which have been developed by pharmaceutical companies and which have been shown to have much greater potency and efficiency than cromoglycate in reducing mast cell histamine release, have *no* effect on asthma [see ✐ p. 362].

    G. False; **ipratropium** can be a useful adjunct to other bronchodilators [see ✐ p. 360 box].

    H. False; **theophylline** is not given by inhalation.

    I. True [see ✐ p. 360 box].

J. True; it could be useful for nocturnal asthma. But note that recent guidelines suggest that long-acting β_2-agonists should be prescribed only for patients already receiving inhaled glucocorticoid therapy.

K. True [see 📖 p. 360].

L. True; sustained-release preparations can result in reasonable plasma concentrations for up to 12 hours [see 📖 p. 361].

M. False [see 📖 Fig. 17.2].

N. False; theophylline, if given i.v., is given slooooooooooowly—over 15–20 minutes.

O. True [see 📖 Fig. 17.3].

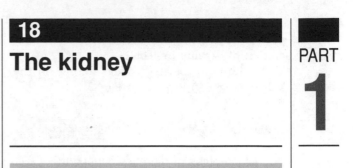

18
The kidney

PART

1

BACKGROUND INFORMATION

The main function of the kidney is the excretion of waste products; it is also important in the regulation of the salt and water content of the body and acid–base balance.

The main active transport mechanism in the renal tubule is the Na^+/K^+-ATPase in the basolateral membrane of the tubule cells. All the constituents of the plasma (other than protein) are filtered into the renal tubules at the glomerulus and 75% of the filtrate is reabsorbed isosmotically in the proximal tubules, bicarbonate in particular. Some organic acids and bases are secreted into the tubule. Water is absorbed in the descending limb of Henle's loop. In the thick ascending limb, which is impermeable to water, there is active reabsorption of salt (this is the major factor in producing hypertonicity in the medulla and thus creating the gradient for the countercurrent concentrating mechanism) via a $Na^+/2Cl^-/K^+$ carrier in the luminal membrane. In the distal tubule, more absorption of Na^+ and Cl^- occurs, and K^+ is secreted into the filtrate. The collecting tubule and ducts have low permeability to both salts and water; here sodium reabsorption and potassium excretion is promoted by **aldosterone** and passive water absorption promoted by the **antidiuretic hormone** (ADH).

Normally less than 1% of filtered sodium is excreted in the urine. Diuretics are drugs which increase sodium (and thus water) excretion by a direct action on the kidney.

Diuretics used clinically are:
- the loop diuretics, e.g. **frusemide**
- thiazides, e.g. **bendrofluazide**
- potassium-sparing diuretics, e.g. **amiloride**, **spironolactone**
- osmotic diuretics, e.g. **mannitol**.

CHAPTER 18

PART

1

Some pharmacological agents can change the pH of the urine. Some drugs can alter the excretion of organic molecules.

A summary chart of drugs acting on the kidney (Fig. 29) is given in Part 2.

QUESTIONS

1. Which class of diuretics causes the greatest excretion of salt and water? Why are they so effective and what is their mechanism of action?

2. Which class of diuretics causes the second most marked excretion of salt and water? What is the mechanism of action?

3. How does **aldosterone** promote Na$^+$ absorption in the distal tubule?

4. Which diuretics cause potassium loss, and which are potassium-sparing? By what mechanism(s) do the latter work and how effective are they as diuretics?

5. Which diuretics promote Ca^{2+} excretion, and which promote Ca^{2+} retention? Which promote Mg^{2+} excretion; which its retention?

6. Which diuretics may exacerbate gout?

7. Which diuretics may cause metabolic alkalosis?

8. What non-renal actions may be seen with:
   a. **thiazides**
   b. **loop diuretics**?

9. Give an example of an osmotic diuretic and explain how it acts.

10. What methods of administration are used with:
    a. **thiazides**
    b. **loop diuretics**
    c. **potassium-sparing diuretics**
    d. **mannitol**?

11. What are the main clinical uses of the diuretics?

12. Indicate which of the following statements are true and which false. If you think a statement is false, explain why.

a. The main pharmacological action of each of the following drugs is due primarily to the unmetabolised parent compound:
A. **frusemide**
B. **ethacrynic acid**
C. **spironolactone**
D. **sodium citrate**
E. **ammonium chloride**.

b. The following drugs are secreted into the proximal tubule:
A. **thiazides**
B. **spironolactone**
C. **frusemide**
D. **mannitol**
E. **triamterene**.

c. These drugs, given orally in the morning, will produce good diuresis but will not interrupt the patients' sleep:
A. **frusemide**
B. **chlorthalidone**
C. **bendrofluazide**
D. **spironolactone**
E. **mannitol**.

ANSWERS

1. Loop diuretics (e.g. **frusemide**) cause the greatest excretion of salt and water. They inhibit salt absorption in the ascending limb of Henle's loop. This reduces the hypertonicity of the medulla which disrupts the kidneys' main countercurrent concentrating mechanism. This in turn means that less ADH-induced water absorption occurs in the collecting tubule. Loop diuretics inhibit

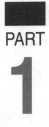

PART

1

the $Na^+/2Cl^-/K^+$ carrier [see 🖉 pp. 373 box, 378 box, Figs 18.5, 18.6, 18.10, 18.11].

2. Thiazides (e.g. **bendrofluazide**) cause the second most marked excretion of salt and water. They inhibit the Na^+/Cl^- co-transporter in the distal tubule [see 🖉 pp. 373 box, 378 box, Figs 18.5, 18.10, 18.13].

3. **Aldosterone** interacts with mineral-corticoid receptors in the distal tubule and directs synthesis of protein mediator(s) which (i) activate Na^+ channels in the luminal membrane and (ii) increase Na^+/K^+-ATPase generation; it also stimulates Na^+/H^+ exchange [see 🖉 p. 372, Fig. 18.14].

4. **Loop diuretics** and **thiazides** cause K^+ loss. **Amiloride**, **triamterene** and **spironolactone** are potassium-sparing; as diuretics they cause only a relatively limited amount of filtered Na^+ to be excreted. Amiloride and triamterene block the aldosterone-controlled Na^+ channels [see Answer 3].

   Spironolactone is a competitive antagonist at the aldosterone receptor [see 🖉 pp. 378 box, 380–381, Figs 18.5, 18.14].

5. **Loop diuretics** promote Ca^{2+} excretion, **thiazides** decrease it. Both loop diuretics and thiazides promote Mg^{2+} excretion [see 🖉 p. 379].

6. **Thiazides**, being organic acids, compete with uric acid for the proximal tubule secretory mechanism; thus they can cause increased plasma uric acid and exacerbate (even precipitate) gout [see 🖉 p. 380].

7. Metabolic alkalosis can result from **loop diuretic** administration, and may be associated with **thiazide**-induced hypokalaemia [see 🖉 p. 378 box].

8. **Thiazides** have some direct vasodilator effects (useful in hypertension) and may also increase blood sugar. **Loop diuretics** may cause vasodilatation

(particularly pulmonary and renal) [see 🖉 pp. 379, 377].

9. **Mannitol** is an osmotic diuretic; it is filtered in the glomerulus and not reabsorbed. It retains water in the tubule and increases the amount of water excreted [see 🖉 p. 382].

10. **a. Thiazides**: oral; **b. Loop diuretics**: oral (i.v. for quick action); **c. K⁺-sparing diuretics**: oral; **d. Mannitol**: i.v.

11. See Figure 12.

12. **a.** Λ. True.

   B. False; the main action, diuresis, is due to adduct formation of **ethacrynic acid** with cysteine [see 🖉 Fig. 18.8].

   C. False; the main action, diuresis, is due to the **spironolactone** metabolite, **canrenone** [see 🖉 p. 380].

   D. False; the main action, alkalinisation of the urine, is due to the fact that the **sodium citrate** is metabolised and the cation is

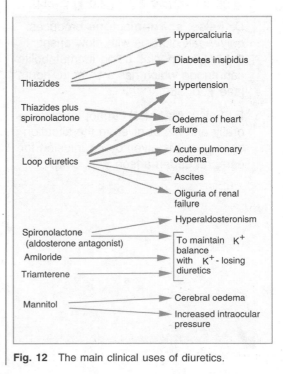

Fig. 12 The main clinical uses of diuretics.

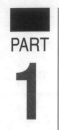

excreted with bicarbonate [see 📖 p. 383 box].

E. False; the main action, acidification of the urine, follows metabolism of **ammonium chloride** [see 📖 p. 383 box].

b. A. True; some is secreted, some filtered in the glomerulus [see 📖 p. 380].

B. False; **spironolactone** is metabolised in the liver and practically none appears in the urine.

C. True [see 📖 p. 378].

D. False; **mannitol** passes into the tubule with the filtrate [see 📖 p. 382].

E. True.

c. A. True; oral **frusemide** acts within 1 hour and its duration of action is 3–6 hours [see 📖 pp. 378–379].

B. and **C.** False; **bendrofluazide** has a duration of action of 12–24 hours and **chlorthalidone** acts for even longer (24–72 hours); with these drugs the patients will need to pass urine during the night [see 📖 p. 380].

D. False; **spironolactone** produces only weak diuresis with slow onset, the active species being its metabolite canrenone which has a $t_{1/2}$ of 16 hours [see 📖 p. 380].

E. False. **Mannitol** cannot be given orally and is not given in the situation specified. It is given by i.v. infusion for cerebral oedema [see 📖 p. 382].

19

The gastrointestinal tract (GIT)

BACKGROUND INFORMATION

Gastric secretion

Acid is secreted from the parietal cells by a proton pump (K^+/H^+-ATPase). Secretion is stimulated by histamine, acetylcholine and gastrin. PGE_2 and PGI_2 inhibit acid secretion and stimulate secretion of mucus and bicarbonate; these actions constitute mucosal protection mechanisms.

It is necessary to reduce acid secretion and/ or to prevent the effects of the acid in patients with peptic ulcer or gastric reflux oesophagitis.

The drugs used clinically are:
- Histamine H_2-receptor antagonists (e.g. **cimetidine**)
- Proton pump inhibitors (e.g. **omeprazole**)
- Antacids (e.g. **magnesium carbonate**)
- Muscarinic-receptor antagonists (e.g. **pirenzepine**)
- Drugs which protect the mucosa (e.g. **sucralfate**)
- Antibacterial agents effective against *Helicobacter pylori*.

A summary chart of drugs used in treatment of peptic ulcer (Fig. 13) is given at the end of this chapter.

Vomiting (emesis)

Emetic stimuli include chemicals in the blood (e.g. **morphine**, endogenous **oestrogens** in pregnancy), and neural input from the labyrinth (motion sickness), from higher CNS centres or from the GIT (various drugs). The chemoreceptor trigger zone is important in integration and the vomiting centre controls the effector mechanisms.

Drugs used clinically are:
- H_1-receptor antagonists (e.g. **meclozine**)

- Muscarinic-receptor antagonists (e.g. **hyoscine**)
- 5-HT$_3$ receptor antagonists (e.g. **ondansetron**)
- Dopamine D$_2$-receptor antagonists (e.g. **metoclopramide** and **phenothiazines**)
- **Cannabinoids**

[see 🖉 p. 395 box].

Motility and expulsion of faeces

Drugs may be used to cause purgation and to treat diarrhoea.

Purgation can be achieved by drugs which:

- increase faecal bulk (e.g. **methylcellulose**)
- increase water content by osmotic action (e.g. **magnesium sulphate**)
- soften the faeces (e.g. **docusate sodium**)
- stimulate motility (e.g. **senna**).

Antidiarrhoeal agents include antimotility agents (e.g. **codeine, loperamide**) and re-hydration solutions.

The pharmacology of bile

The main pathological condition is cholesterol gallstones. Surgery is the treatment of choice but primary bile acids (e.g. **chenodeoxycholic acid**) can dissolve non-calcified cholesterol gall-stones. Drugs are also used to relax biliary spasm.

QUESTIONS

1. How is acid secretion from parietal cells controlled? What intracellular transduction mechanisms are involved?

2. Which is the main group of drugs used to reduce gastric acid secretion? Give examples of this and other groups. What are the mechanisms of action?

3. Which drugs are sometimes used as adjuncts to the main agents used to reduce acid secretion? Give examples. What is the mechanism of action?

4. What important drug interactions occur with **H$_2$-receptor antagonists**?

5. What is **misoprostol** and what actions underlie its useful clinical actions?

6. Drugs **a.** .... and **b.** .... are cytoprotective, acting by coating peptic ulcers. **b.** also has another action, **c.** .... , which is useful in peptic ulcer therapy.

7. Which neurotransmitters are involved in the reflex pathways controlling vomiting? Which receptors do they act on?

8. What anti-emetic drug(s) are useful for motion sickness?

9. What anti-emetic drug(s) would be useful in vomiting due to the anticancer drug **cisplatin**?

10. What drugs could be used to control morning sickness during pregnancy?

11. Which laxative(s) might be considered to be agents of choice in preventing constipation? Which for prompt purgation?

12. What drug would you use for symptomatic treatment of constipation in a patient with painful rectal haemorrhoids (piles)?

13. If drugs are necessary to treat traveller's diarrhoea, what agents could be used?

14. What oral rehydration agents could be used in the treatment of **a.** severe diarrhoea in infants; **b.** moderate but continued diarrhoea in adults.

15. Drugs **a.** .... or **b.** .... could be used to dissolve non-calcified cholesterol gallstones.

16. **a.** What agents could be used to treat biliary spasm?

    b. What agents could make matters worse?

17. Infection with microorganism **a.** .... is thought to play a part in the development of peptic ulcer.

    b. What agents are used to treat infection with this microorganism?

18. Indicate which of the following statements are true and which false. If you think a statement is false, explain why.

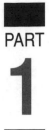

PART

1

65

A. Gastric acid secretion is controlled by **gastrin**.

B. Dicyclomine has antispasmodic action in the GIT by virtue of antagonising the action of acetylcholine on muscarinic M_3-receptors on smooth muscle.

C. Aluminium hydroxide is an effective antacid but continued use of this agent can cause constipation.

D. Magnesium hydroxide is an effective antacid but can cause constipation.

E. Pirenzepine, a muscarinic-receptor antagonist, is not useful for reducing gastric acid secretion because it has marked side effects on the heart (tachycardia) and the CNS (stimulation).

F. Ondansetron has an anti-emetic effect by action on $5-HT_3$ receptors.

G. Hyoscine is useful for the treatment of motion sickness once it starts but is less useful in preventing it.

H. Loperamide is an 'antimotility agent' used to treat diarrhoea.

I. The chemoreceptor trigger zone can be stimulated by agents which do not cross into the CSF since it lies outside the blood–brain barrier.

J. Cimetidine has potent inhibitory effects on gastric acid secretion by stimulating histamine H_2-receptors on gastric parietal cells.

ANSWERS

1. See Figure 13 on page 67.

2. The H_2-receptor antagonists, e.g. **cimetidine, ranitidine**. They act by competitive antagonism at the H_2-receptor on the parietal cell. They are the drugs of choice for peptic ulcer treatment. Muscarinic-receptor antagonists (competitive antagonists at M_1-receptors, e.g. **pirenzepine**) are alternative drugs. Proton-pump inhibitors (e.g.

omeprazole) are also valuable [see 📖 Figs 19.1, 19.2, 19.3].

3. Antacids (e.g. **magnesium trisilicate, aluminium hydroxide**) are often used as adjuncts to H_2-receptor antagonists to provide supplementary relief of symptoms. These drugs directly neutralise the acid [see 📖 p. 391].

4. **Cimetidine** (but not the other H_2-antagonists) inhibits cytochrome P-450 and retards metabolism of the many drugs metabolised by the mixed function oxidases [see 📖 p. 390].

5. **Misoprostol** is a stable analogue of PGE_2. It inhibits histamine-stimulated gastric acid secretion and also increases bicarbonate and mucus secretion [see 📖 p. 393, Fig.19.2].

6. **a. Sucralfate; b. tripotassium dicitratobismuthate; c.** this latter agent also adsorbs pepsin [see 📖 p. 392].

7. **5-HT** on $5-HT_3$ receptors, **dopamine** on D_2-receptors, **histamine** on H_1-receptors, **acetylcholine** on muscarinic receptors [see 📖 p. 397 box, Fig. 19.8].

8. H_1-receptor antagonists (e.g. **meclozine, cinnarizine, cyclizine**) and muscarinic-receptor antagonists (e.g. **hyoscine**) are useful in motion sickness, the latter mainly for prevention [see 📖 p. 397 box].

9. The $5-HT_3$ receptor antagonist, **ondansetron**, is effective against cisplatin-induced vomiting; other drugs used are the phenothiazines (e.g. **thiethylperazine**) and dopamine D_2-antagonists (**metoclopramide, domperidone**) [see 📖 pp. 395–396].

10. No drugs should be given, if possible. For serious vomiting (hyperemesis gravidarum), the phenothiazine, **thiethylperazine**, could be used, with *circumspection* [see 📖 p. 395 box].

11. A diet rich in fibre is best for preventing constipation. If drugs are necessary, the **bulk laxatives** are probably nearest in action to this. **Senna** causes prompt purgation [see 📖 p. 400 box].

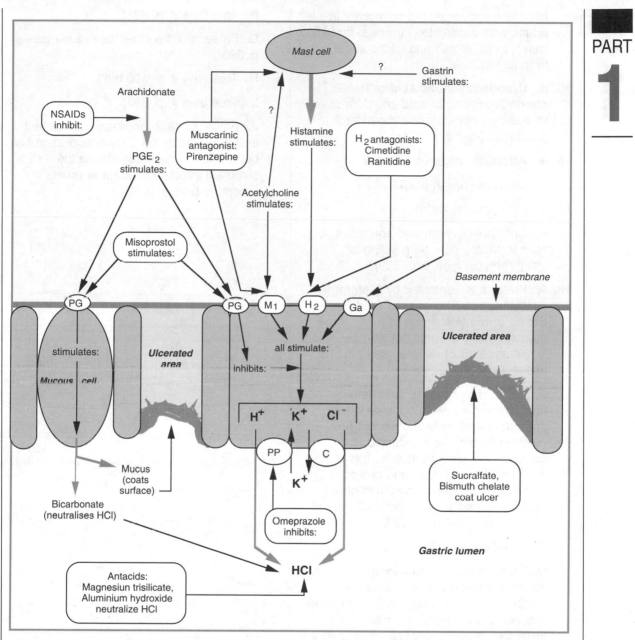

Fig. 13 Diagram of gastric mucosa showing the processes involved in acid secretion, the transmitters/mediators controlling these processes and the sites of action of drugs which could be used in the treatment of peptic ulcer (shown in boxes). The ulcerated area is depicted schematically. NSAIDs increase acid secretion. The receptors shown are H = histamine, M = muscarinic, PG = prostaglandin E_2 (the EP_3 receptor), Ga = gastrin, PP = proton pump, C = co-transporter.

12. A faecal softener, e.g. **dioctyl sodium sulphosuccinate**, or a saline purgative used with moderation [see 📖 p. 400 box].

13. **Loperamide** or **codeine** or **diphenoxylate**. Chemotherapy is seldom necessary [see 📖 p. 399].

14. **a.** Isotonic solutions containing both sodium and glucose, made up from sachets of Oral Rehydration Salts Formula C (WHO) can be life-saving in serious diarrhoea in malnourished infants [see 📖 p. 400 box].

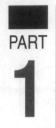

b. If oral rehydration is necessary in adults with moderate diarrhoea, fruit juice with a pinch of salt and a little sugar will probably suffice.

15. a. Ursodeoxycholic acid or **b. chenodeoxycholic acid** could be used to dissolve non-calcified cholesterol gallstones [see 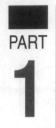 p. 401].

16. a. Atropine, **organic nitrates**.

b. Opiates [see 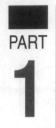 p. 401].

17. a. *Helicobacter pylori*.

b. Colloidal bismuth and antibiotics, e.g. metronidazole plus tetracycline or clarithromycin [see 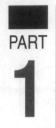 p. 389].

18. A. False; it is controlled by **histamine**, **acetylcholine** and **gastrin** (and the details of the interaction of these three mediators in the control of acid secretion is still a matter of debate) [see Fig. 13 and 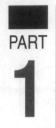 Fig. 19.2].

B. False; **dicyclomine** does have antispasmodic action in the GIT but, perhaps surprisingly, it does not have much effect on the muscarinic M_3-receptors on smooth muscle. It is more active on M_1-receptors and probably affects GIT motility by an effect on autonomic and enteric neuronal control mechanisms [see 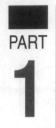 p. 128, Table 6.1].

C. True [see 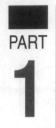 p. 391].

D. False; **magnesium hydroxide** is an effective antacid but, like other magnesium salts (magnesium carbonate, magnesium sulphate and magnesium trisilicate), it has a laxative effect [see 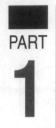 p. 391].

E. False; **pirenzepine** reduces gastric acid secretion by an action on the M_1-receptors on the postsynaptic membrane at parasympathetic ganglia and also, probably, on the M_1-receptors on gastric parietal cells; but it has little or no effect on the cardiac M_2-receptors and does not penetrate the CNS; so it will not have marked side effects on these tissues [see 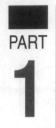 p. 391].

F. True [see 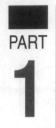 p. 396].

G. False; it is the other way round [see 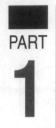 p. 395].

H. True [see 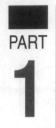 p. 400 box].

I. True [see 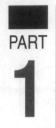 p. 393].

J. False; **cimetidine** does have potent inhibitory effects on gastric acid secretion but it does so by antagonising the stimulant effect of **histamine** on H_2-receptors [see 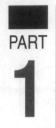 p. 389].

20

The endocrine pancreas and the control of blood glucose

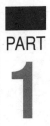

BACKGROUND INFORMATION

The islets of Langerhans in the pancreas secrete **insulin** from β-cells and **glucagon** from α_2-cells. The plasma glucose level is the main factor determining insulin secretion.

Insulin is a 'fuel storage' hormone; it increases glucose uptake and glycogen synthesis by cells and decreases glycogen breakdown and gluconeogenesis, the result being a decrease in blood glucose.

Glucagon is a fuel-mobilising hormone; it stimulates gluconeogenesis, glycogenolysis and lipolysis, the result being an increase in blood sugar. **Growth hormone, glucocorticoids** and **catecholamines** also increase blood glucose.

The main disorder of blood glucose control is diabetes mellitus, of which there are two forms: insulin-dependent (juvenile onset) diabetes and non-insulin-dependent (maturity onset) diabetes.

The main drugs used clinically are:
Insulin (given by injection) and the **sulphonylureas** (e.g. tolbutamide) and biguanides; these last two are given orally.

QUESTIONS

1. What are the actions of **insulin** on:
   a. carbohydrate metabolism; **b.** fat metabolism; **c.** protein metabolism?

2. What form of **insulin** is used in emergency, e.g. in ketoacidosis?

3. Name an intermediate-action **insulin** preparation.

4. What is the commonest and most serious complication of **insulin** treatment? How is it treated?

5. What **sulphonylurea agent** is a safe drug and is least likely to cause hypoglycaemia?

6. What is the mechanism of action of **metformin**? What is its main role in the treatment of diabetes?

7. Indicate which of the following statements are true and which false. If you think a statement is false, explain why.

   A. Insulin binds to intracellular receptors.

   B. Sulphonylurea drugs stimulate insulin secretion from β-cells in the pancreas and are thus only effective in diabetics with functioning β-cells.

   C. Sulphonylurea drugs increase the potassium permeability of β-cells by facilitating the activation of the ATP-sensitive potassium channels.

   D. Acarbose interferes with the uptake of glucose into the β-cell.

   E. Insulin is a polypeptide with a molecular weight of approximately 6000.

   F. Catecholamines increase insulin release by an action on α_2-adrenoceptors.

   G. Amylin, released from β-cells with insulin, will also lower the blood glucose concentration.

ANSWERS

1. **a.** It increases glucose uptake into cells and glycogen synthesis and decreases glycogen breakdown and gluconeogenesis.

   b. It increases synthesis of triglycerides and fatty acids and decreases lipolysis.

   c. It decreases protein breakdown and increases amino-acid uptake and protein synthesis [see ✎ Table 20.1].

2. **Soluble insulin** given in low doses by i.v. infusion [see ✎ Table 20.3].

3. Isophane insulin; insulin zinc suspension (amorphous) [see ✎ Table 20.3].

4. Hypoglycaemia is the main undesirable effect of **insulin** treatment; it is treated with oral glucose, or, in emergency, intravenous glucose or glucagon intramuscularly [see ✎ p. 413].

5. Tolbutamide [see ✎ Table 20.4].

6. It increases glucose uptake by cells (if some insulin is present); it is used with sulphonylureas, if these have ceased to work effectively [see ✎ p. 411 box].

7. A. False; the **insulin** receptor is on the surface of the cell membrane [see ✎ Fig. 20.3].

B. True [see ✎ p. 411 box].

C. False; they reduce the potassium permeability by blocking the ATP-sensitive potassium channels. ATP normally closes this channel, decreasing potassium permeability and causing the cell to depolarise; this results in Ca^{2+} entry and insulin secretion. The sulphonylurea drugs mimic the effect of ATP [see ✎ p. 415].

D. False; **acarbose**, an α-glucosidase inhibitor, reduces the absorption of carbohydrate from the intestine [see ✎ p. 416].

E. True [see ✎ p. 404].

F. False; α$_2$-adrenoceptor activation *inhibits* insulin release [see ✎ p. 404].

G. False; amylin may *elevate* the blood glucose concentration, but whether this is physiologically important has yet to be determined [see ✎ p. 408].

21
The endocrine system

BACKGROUND INFORMATION

The anterior pituitary
The anterior pituitary, under the influence of various releasing factors from the hypothalamus, secretes a series of regulatory hormones which act on target organs such as the adrenal cortex, the thyroid, the ovary and mammary gland, and the liver and other peripheral tissues. Most of these target organs in turn release peripheral hormones, some of which have negative feedback effects on the hypothalamus.

Drugs used clinically are: growth hormone-releasing factor, growth hormone (GH), **analogues of GH, protirelin** (thyrotrophin-releasing factor), **octreotide** (somatostatin analogue), **corticotrophin-releasing factor, gonadorelin** [see Ch. 22].

The posterior pituitary
The posterior pituitary secretes:
- **oxytocin** (a uterine spasmogen)
- the antidiuretic hormone (ADH, **vasopressin**).

Drugs used clinically are: vasopressin and an analogue, **desmopressin**, and **oxytocin** (this last is used in obstetrics).

The thyroid
Synthesis of the thyroid hormones, **thyroxine** (T$_4$) and **triiodothyronine** (T$_3$), involves iodination of tyrosine residues on the thyroglobulin molecules within the lumen of the thyroid follicle. The iodinated thyroglobulin is then endocytosed and broken down, and T$_4$ and T$_3$ are released. Synthesis and secretion are controlled by thyrotrophin and influenced by plasma iodide. Abnormalities of thyroid function include hyperthyroidism (either diffuse toxic goitre or toxic nodular goitre), simple non-toxic goitre (which

is due to dietary iodine deficiency) and hypo-thyroidism.

The main drugs used clinically are:
- thioureylenes (e.g. **propylthiouracil**), **radioiodine, iodide**; these are used in hyperthyroidism
- **thyroxine** (T_4), **triiodothyronine** (T_3); these are used in hypothyroidism.

Figure 14 is a summary chart of agents affecting the thyroid and the action of the thyroid hormones.

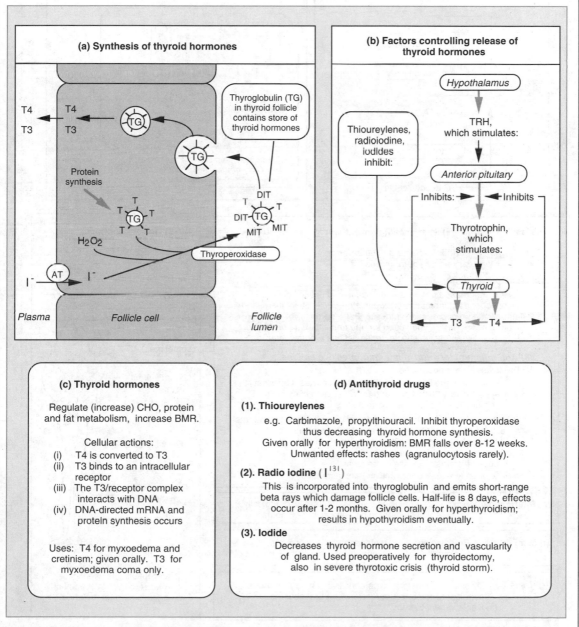

Fig. 14 Chart of thyroid function showing (a) synthesis of thyroid hormones; (b) factors controlling their release, actions, mechanism of actions and uses of: (c) thyroid hormones and (d) antithyroid dugs. AT = active transport; TG = thyroglobulin; CHO = carbohydrate; TRH = thyroid-releasing hormone; DIT = diiodotyrosine; MIT = monoiodotyrosine.

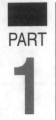

Corticotrophin and adrenal steroids

Corticotrophin (ACTH) stimulates synthesis and release of glucocorticoids from the adrenal cortex. Corticotrophin release from the anterior pituitary is regulated by the hypothalamic corticotrophin-releasing factor which in turn is regulated by neural factors and the negative-feedback effects of plasma glucocorticoids.

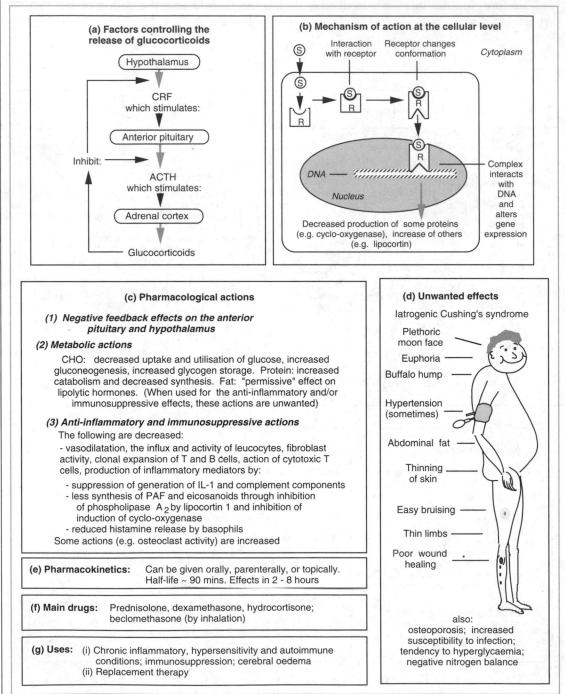

(a) Factors controlling the release of glucocorticoids

Hypothalamus → CRF which stimulates: → Anterior pituitary → ACTH which stimulates: → Adrenal cortex → Glucocorticoids

Inhibit:

(b) Mechanism of action at the cellular level

Interaction with receptor — Receptor changes conformation — *Cytoplasm*

DNA — *Nucleus*

Complex interacts with DNA and alters gene expression

Decreased production of some proteins (e.g. cyclo-oxygenase), increase of others (e.g. lipocortin)

(c) Pharmacological actions

(1) Negative feedback effects on the anterior pituitary and hypothalamus

(2) Metabolic actions

CHO: decreased uptake and utilisation of glucose, increased gluconeogenesis, increased glycogen storage. Protein: increased catabolism and decreased synthesis. Fat: "permissive" effect on lipolytic hormones. (When used for the anti-inflammatory and/or immunosuppressive effects, these actions are unwanted)

(3) Anti-inflammatory and immunosuppressive actions

The following are decreased:
- vasodilatation, the influx and activity of leucocytes, fibroblast activity, clonal expansion of T and B cells, action of cytotoxic T cells, production of inflammatory mediators by:

  - suppression of generation of IL-1 and complement components
  - less synthesis of PAF and eicosanoids through inhibition of phospholipase A_2 by lipocortin 1 and inhibition of induction of cyclo-oxygenase
  - reduced histamine release by basophils
Some actions (e.g. osteoclast activity) are increased

(e) Pharmacokinetics: Can be given orally, parenterally, or topically. Half-life ~ 90 mins. Effects in 2 - 8 hours

(f) Main drugs: Prednisolone, dexamethasone, hydrocortisone; beclomethasone (by inhalation)

(g) Uses: (i) Chronic inflammatory, hypersensitivity and autoimmune conditions; immunosuppression; cerebral oedema
(ii) Replacement therapy

(d) Unwanted effects

Iatrogenic Cushing's syndrome

Plethoric moon face

Euphoria

Buffalo hump

Hypertension (sometimes)

Abdominal fat

Thinning of skin

Easy bruising

Thin limbs

Poor wound healing

also: osteoporosis; increased susceptibility to infection; tendency to hyperglycaemia; negative nitrogen balance

Fig. 15 Chart of the glucocorticoids showing (a) factors controlling release; (b) the mechanism of action at the cellular level; (c) the pharmacological actions; (d) unwanted effects; (e) pharmacokinetic factors; (f) the main drugs; and (g) clinical uses. S = steroid; R = steroid receptor; CRF = corticotrophin-releasing factor; CHO = carbohydrate.

The **glucocorticoids** have three types of action:

1. metabolic
2. regulatory (see negative-feedback above)
3. anti-inflammatory and immunosuppressive.

Drugs used clinically include:

- glucocorticoids (e.g. **hydrocortisone, prednisolone, dexamethasone**)
- **tetracosactrin**, a synthetic analogue of corticotrophin (infrequently used).

Endocrinologists tend to emphasise mainly the metabolic actions of the glucocorticoids, but the most common and general use of these drugs is for their anti-inflammatory/immunosuppressive actions. Used for these latter actions, the glucocorticoids are said to be responsible for more iatrogenic* disease (i.e. disease caused by the doctor) than any other group of drugs. When they were first introduced they produced profound improvement in many chronic inflammatory conditions, but not long afterwards it was said by a perspicacious clinician that the improvement enabled a patient to proceed unaided to the post-mortem room. It is surprising that these drugs are usually rather neglected in pharmacology courses.

Figure 15 is a chart of the ACTH–glucocorticoid axis and the drugs affecting it.

Mineralocorticoids

The release of mineralocorticoids from the adrenal cortex is controlled by the renin–angiotensin system. The main hormone is **aldosterone**; its main effect is to cause sodium retention in the kidney.

The drug used clinically is **fludrocortisone**, given orally with a glucocorticoid in replacement therapy.

Parathyroid hormone, vitamin D, bone mineral homeostasis

The members of the vitamin D family are true hormones. Precursors are converted to **calcifediol** (25,hydroxyvitamin D_3) in the liver, then to the main hormone, **calcitriol**, (1,25,dihydroxyvitamin D_3) in the kidney.

---

* According to some classicists, the correct term should be 'iatrogenous'.

Calcitriol increases plasma calcium by mobilising it from bone, increasing its absorption in the intestine and decreasing its excretion by the kidney. **Parathyroid hormone** increases blood calcium by mobilising calcium from bone and increasing calcitriol synthesis in the kidney.

The drugs used clinically are: ergocalciferol (a vitamin D precursor), **calcitriol, disodium etidronate, calcitonin**.

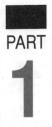

QUESTIONS

The hypothalamus and the pituitary glands

1. What are the two principal actions of **ADH**? On which receptor does it act?

2. **a.** .... can be used to suppress lactation because of its action on the anterior pituitary because **b.** ....

3. How is **desmopressin** administered? What is its principal clinical use? Is it superior to **vasopressin** when used for this purpose?

The thyroid

4. What is the mechanism of action of the thioureylene drugs?

5. **a.** What are the main effects of T_4?

   b. What is its mechanism of action at the cellular level?

6. How long does it take for the peak clinical response to occur with **a. carbimazole; b. T_3; c. T_4?**

7. **Propylthiouracil** is used to treat hyperthyroidism. It is given orally and produces 90% reduction in thyroid hormone synthesis within 12 hours. However, its full clinical response usually takes many weeks to develop. Why?

8. **a.** .... on injection, causes a rapid increase in thyrotrophin in the blood of normal patients and can be used to test thyroid function. Its mechanism of action is **b.** ....

73

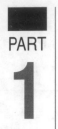

PART

1

9. What is the action and mechanism of action of high doses of **iodide** in hyperthyroidism?

ACTH and the adrenal steroids

10. **a.** What are the metabolic actions of the **glucocorticoids**?

    b. In what circumstances might these be necessary?

    c. In what circumstances might they be unwanted?

11. What are the main unwanted effects of prolonged **glucocorticoid** excess?

12. What is the intracellular mechanism of action of the **glucocorticoids**?

13. What actions of the **glucorticoids** are useful when they are used for anti-inflammatory/immunosuppressive effects?

14. What mechanisms of action underlie the anti-inflammatory effects of the **glucocorticoids**?

15. **a.** What corticosteroid is the drug of choice for systemic anti-inflammatory actions?

    b. Which corticosteroid(s) can be used topically in aerosol form?

    c. Which are inactive until converted in vivo?

    d. Which glucocorticoid is the drug of choice for replacement therapy?

16. What is the common unwanted effect experienced by patients taking a **glucocorticoid** aerosol for asthma?

17. **a.** What are the main actions of **tetracosactrin**?

    b. What is it used for?

18. What is the intracellular mechanism of action of **fludrocortisone**?

19. What potential hazard, related to the regulatory actions of the **glucocorticoids**, must be kept in mind

after prolonged therapy with these agents?

Parathyroid hormone, vitamin D and bone mineral homeostasis

20. Which vitamin D preparation is most potent in regulating plasma $[Ca^{2+}]$?

21. What are the principal clinical uses of **vitamin D**? Which preparations are used?

22. Indicate which of the following statements are true and which false. If you think a statement is false, explain why.

    A. Both **insulin** and **thyroid hormone** (T_4) bind to intracellular receptors.

    B. **Vasopressin** causes contraction of vascular smooth muscle by an action on V_2-receptors.

    C. T_4 has a more rapid and shorter-lasting effect on basal metabolic rate than T_3.

    D. **Fludrocortisone** has to be given i.m.

    E. **Catecholamines** cause increased glycogenolysis and decreased glucose uptake and thus tend to oppose the actions of insulin.

    F. **Radioiodine** can be used for the treatment of thyrotoxicosis, but it is likely to cause hypothyroidism eventually.

    G. Either **thyroxine** (T_4) or **liothyronine** (T_3) can be used for replacement therapy in hypothyroidism.

    H. The thioureylene drugs (e.g. **carbimazole**) have antithyroid action by virtue of preventing the action of thyroid-stimulating hormone on the thyroid.

    I. The full clinical response to **carbimazole** may take weeks or even months to develop.

    J. **Betamethasone** is a glucocorticoid only used topically and as an aerosol.

ANSWERS

The hypothalamus and the pituitary glands

1. It increases water reabsorption (V_1-receptors) and causes vasoconstriction (V_2-receptors) [see 📖 p. 424 box].

2. **a. Bromocryptine** can suppress lactation because **b.** it is a dopamine agonist and inhibits prolactin secretion from the anterior pituitary [see 📖 Fig. 21.3].

3. **Desmopressin** is usually given intranasally and is used to treat diabetes insipidus. It is superior to **vasopressin** for this purpose since it has less vasoconstrictor effect and a longer duration of action [see 📖 p. 425].

The thyroid

4. The thioureylene drugs **carbimazole**, **propylthiouracil**, **methimazole** block the organification of iodine [see 📖 p. 432 box, Fig 21.5].

5. **a.** It stimulates metabolism causing increased O_2 consumption and metabolic rate; It influences growth and development [see 📖 p. 430 box].

   b. It enters cells, is converted to T_3 which binds to a receptor; this interacts with DNA leading to mRNA and protein synthesis [see 📖 p. 429].

6. **a. Carbimazole**: 2–3 months; **b. T_4**: 6–8 days; **c. T_3**: 12–24 hours [see 📖 Figs 21.9, 21.12].

7. **Propylthiouracil** acts by preventing iodination of tyrosine residues, but the thyroid has large stores of T_4 and T_3 already synthesised by previous iodination of tyrosine residues in the thyroglobulin within the thyroid follicles [see 📖 Fig. 21.5, p. 431].

8. **a. Protirelin; b.** stimulation of the anterior pituitary [see 📖 pp. 420, 428, Fig 21.8].

9. It transiently decreases T_3 and T_4 secretion and reduces thyroid vascularity [see 📖 pp. 432, 432 box, Figs 21.5, 21.8].

ACTH and the adrenal steroids

10. **a.** See Figure 15 (p. 72).

    b. The metabolic actions are required when **glucocorticoids** are used for replacement therapy.

    c. The metabolic actions are unwanted when glucocorticoids are used for their anti-inflammatory/immunosuppressive effects [see 📖 p. 434 box].

11. Iatrogenic Cushing's syndrome and suppression of endogenous glucocorticoid synthesis [for details and other effects, see Fig. 15 and 📖 pp. 441, 442 box, Fig. 21.16].

12. The intracellular ligand/receptor complex interacts with DNA and modifies gene transcription—inducing synthesis of some proteins and inhibiting synthesis of others [see Fig. 15 and 📖 Fig. 21.15, p. 441 box].

13. See Figure 15 and 📖 p. 438 box, Figs 11.3, 11.4, 11.5, 17.3.

14. Anti-inflammatory effects are produced by two mechanisms:

    • decreased generation of some inflammatory mediators due either to direct inhibition of transcription (e.g. of cyclo-oxygenase) and/or interference with the intracellular transduction mechanisms for their production

    • generation of anti-inflammatory mediators such as lipocortin-1 [see 📖 pp. 439–441, 441 box].

15. **a. Prednisolone; b. beclomethasone; c. cortisone, prednisone; d. hydrocortisone** [see 📖 Table 21.2]. Note that hydrocortisone must be teamed with a mineralocorticoid for replacement therapy.

16. Oral thrush can occur with **inhaled glucocorticoids**, and frequently does [see 📖 p. 363 box].

PART

1

17. a. It stimulates synthesis and release of glucocorticoids and has a trophic action on adrenal cortical cells [see p. 443].

b. The diagnosis of adrenal cortical insufficiency. These drugs are now rarely, if ever, used for anti-inflammatory therapy [see 📖 p. 444].

18. Like aldosterone it binds to intracellular receptors in target organs; the complex initiates DNA-directed synthesis of mRNA and mediator proteins [see 📖 Figs 18.5, 18.14, 21.15].

19. The negative-feedback action of glucocorticoids results in suppression of the patient's capacity to synthesise endogenous corticosteroids. Sudden withdrawal of therapy can result in acute adrenal insufficiency. Note that the more prolonged the therapy, the slower the withdrawal must be, i.e. the more gradual the reduction in dose.

Parathyroid hormone, vitamin D, bone mineral homeostasis

20. Calcitriol [see 📖 p. 449].

21. To prevent and treat vitamin D deficiency (rickets, osteomalacia, intestinal malabsorption, liver disease) and the hypocalcaemia of hypoparathyroidism: **ergocalciferol**, **dihydrotachysterol**. To treat the bone disorder of renal disease: **calcitriol** [see 📖 p. 450 box].

22. A. False; **thyroid hormone** does bind to an intracellular receptor but the **insulin** receptor is on the surface of the cell membrane [see 📖 Fig. 20.3].

B. False; the statement would be fine if 'V$_1$' was substituted for 'V$_2$'. V$_2$-receptors occur on renal tubule cells [see 📖 p. 424 box].

C. False; it's the other way round [see 📖 Fig. 21.9].

D. False; this is true for **aldosterone**. **Fludrocortisone** can be given orally [see 📖 p. 445 box].

E. True [see 📖 Table 20.2].

F. True [see 📖 p. 432 box].

G. False; T$_4$ (but not T$_3$) is used for replacement therapy. T$_3$ is used only for myxoedema coma [see 📖 p. 433].

H. False; they inhibit thyroid hormone synthesis; they block the iodination of tyrosine residues within the thyroglobulin molecule by inhibiting thyroperoxidase action [see 📖 Figs 21.5, 21.11].

I. True [see 📖 Fig. 21.12].

J. False; this statement is true for **beclomethasone** and **budesonide**; betamethasone is given orally, or parenterally. It is a real nuisance that these names sound so similar but that's the way it is; just grit your teeth and bear it [see 📖 Table 21.2].

22

The reproductive system

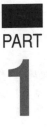

BACKGROUND INFORMATION

The female and male reproductive systems

Hypothalamic anterior pituitary and ovarian hormones control the development of the reproductive organs and secondary sexual characteristics. In the female, with the onset of puberty, these hormones control the menstrual cycle and have a significant role in pregnancy.

The menstrual cycle

At the start of the menstrual cycle, hypothalamic gonadotrophin-releasing hormone (GnRH) stimulates the anterior pituitary to release follicle-stimulating hormone (FSH) and luteinising hormone (LH), which act on the ovary. FSH controls follicle development and is the main hormone regulating oestrogen secretion. LH stimulates ovulation at midcycle and is the main hormone controlling progesterone secretion from the corpus luteum. Oestrogen controls the proliferative phase of the uterine endometrium, progesterone the later, secondary phase and both have negative-feedback effects on the hypothalamus and anterior pituitary thus modulating their own secretion. If a fertilised ovum is implanted, the corpus luteum continues to secrete progesterone (the main pregnancy hormone) during the pregnancy.

The main drugs used clinically are:

Oestrogen, e.g. **ethinyl oestradiol**
Progestogens, e.g. **hydroxyprogesterone hexanoate, norethisterone**
Gonadotrophin-releasing hormones, e.g. **gonadorelin.**

Others are:
Anti-oestrogens, e.g. **tamoxifen** (used for breast cancer), **clomiphene** (this inhibits only negative-feedback actions)

Antiprogestogens, e.g. **mifepristone** (acts mainly on uterus), **danazol** (inhibits negative-feedback actions).

A non-therapeutic use of oestrogens and progestogens is for oral contraception. It is important to know the unwanted effects and the potential beneficial effects of oral contraceptives [see 📖 pp. 467–469].

Sex hormones in the male

Hypothalamic GnRH stimulates the anterior pituitary to release both FSH, which controls gametogenesis in the testis, and LH (also called interstitial-cell-stimulating hormone, ICSH) which regulates testosterone secretion from the interstitial cells of the testis.

Drugs used clinically are:

Androgens, e.g. **testosterone, mesterolone**
Anti-androgens, e.g. **cyproterone acetate, finasteride**
Anabolic steroids, e.g. **nandrolone**.

The uterus

Uterine function (particularly as regards the state of the endometrium) is under the control of the sex steroids which in turn are regulated by hypothalamic and anterior pituitary hormones. During and after parturition, posterior pituitary hormones have a role in controlling the myometrium.

Drugs used clinically are:

Oxytoxic agents, e.g. **oxytocin, ergometrine**
Analogues of E or F type prostaglandins, e.g. **dinoprostone**
Uterine relaxants, e.g. the β_2-adrenoceptor agonist, **terbutaline**.

QUESTIONS

1. List the main uses of **oestrogens** other than for contraception.

2. What are the two main types of preparation used for oral contraception in the female? What are the differences in administration? What are the relative advantages of each? How does each type of preparation work?

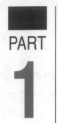

PART

1

3. What is the mechanism of action of the **sex steroids** at the cellular level? What hormonal factors influence the expression of oestrogen and progestogen receptors?

4. What drugs can induce ovulation and how do they work?

5. What are the advantages and disadvantages of using **oestrogens** for postmenopausal hormone replacement therapy?

6. What is the main hazard of oral contraception with the combination pill?

7. In a sexually-active woman, missing a dose of the .... pill could result in pregnancy. Explain why.

8. Name some **oestrogen** and **progestogen** preparations used in combination contraceptive pills.

9. What **testosterone** preparation can be given orally?

10. What drug can effectively relieve spasmodic dysmenorrhoea? Explain how.

11. What agents can cause increased tone and/or contractions of the myometrium?

12. Indicate which of the following statements are true and which false. If you think a statement is false, explain why.

A. **Stilboestrol** is used mainly in the therapy of cancer.

B. **Danazol** inhibits the midcycle surge of **gonadotrophins** in the female.

C. **Clomiphene** binds to progesterone receptors in the hypothalamus and anterior pituitary.

D. There are two main groups of **progestogens**:

(i) **progesterone-like**, and

(ii) **testosterone** derivatives.

E. **Anabolic steroids** can increase athletic performance without significant physiological hazard.

F. **Gonadorelin**, given continuously in females, stimulates gonadotrophin release.

G. An extract of the urine of postmenopausal women is used to treat infertility.

H. β_2-**adrenoceptor antagonists** are used to relax the uterus in prevention of premature labour.

I. **Prostaglandin E$_2$** analogues cause increased tone and contraction of uterine muscle.

J. **Prostaglandin E$_1$** analogues relax cervical muscles.

K. All **oestrogen** preparations given orally will undergo some degree of first-pass metabolism.

L. **Finasteride** inhibits 5α-reductase which converts dihydrotestosterone to testosterone.

M. **Finasteride** is used to treat non-malignant prostate hyperplasia.

ANSWERS

1. Replacement therapy, treatment of certain cancers, vaginitis (topical oestrogen), acne, menstrual disorders [see 📖 p. 459 box].

2. The two types of oral contraceptives are:

- combinations of an **oestrogen** with a **progestogen**, taken 21 days followed by 7 pill-free days

- **progestogen** alone, taken continuously.

The combination pill is the most effective form of oral contraception. The **oestrogen** inhibits FSH release, and therefore follicle development. The **progestogen** inhibits LH release, and therefore ovulation, and makes cervical mucus inhospitable to sperm. Together they render the endometrium unsuitable for ovum implantation.

The progestogen-only pill can be useful after childbirth since, lacking oestrogen, it does not interfere with lactation. The main action is on the cervical mucus [see 📖 pp. 467–469].

3. All steroids bind to intracellular receptors; the complex then initiates DNA-directed RNA and protein synthesis. There may also be repression of expression of certain genes [see 📖 p. 458, also Figs 2.3, 21.15]. Sex steroid receptors are present only in the reproductive and secondary sex tissues. **Oestrogens** induce the synthesis of **progestogen** receptors. Progesterone decreases oestrogen receptor expression. **Prolactin** increases oestrogen receptors in the mammary gland but not in the uterus [see 📖 p. 458].

4. Drugs which induce ovulation include **clomiphene** and **cyclofenil**, also the gonadotrophin-releasing hormones when given in pulsatile fashion [see 📖 pp. 460, 466, 466 box, Fig. 22.6].

5. Given cyclically during and after the menopause, **oestrogens** (in low dose) can relieve symptoms such as hot flushes, sweating, and atrophic vaginitis and decrease the risk of osteoporosis. They may also reduce the incidence of myocardial infarction and stroke. There can be an increased risk of gall bladder disease, hypertension and endometrial cancer. The last condition is less likely if a **progestogen** is also given cyclically but this may counteract the protective effect of the oestrogens against myocardial infarction and stroke. A slightly increased risk of breast cancer is reported. Oestrogens commonly cause postmenopausal bleeding (which must be differentiated from bleeding due to endo-metrial cancer) [see 📖 pp. 461–462].

6. An increased risk of thrombo-embolic disease if other risk factors (e.g. smoking, hypertension) are present [see 📖 pp. 467–468].

7. Missing a dose of the **progestogen-only** pill could result in pregnancy because the contraceptive effect of this preparation is less reliable; in particular, the decreased level of progestogen after a missed pill could mean that ovulation is not inhibited [see 📖 p. 468].

8. Oestrogen: usually **ethinyloestradiol**. Progestogen: **norethisterone** or **levonorgestrel** (others are desogestrel, ethinodiol, gestodene).

9. **Mesterolone** is a testosterone preparation which can be given orally [see 📖 p. 464].

10. **NSAIDs** can relieve spasmodic dysmenorrhoea since the spasm is due mainly to increased generation of PGE_2 and $PGF_2\alpha$; NSAIDs, by inhibiting cyclo-oxygenase, interfere with prostaglandin generation [see 📖 pp. 472–473].

11. **Oxytocin**, **ergometrine**, **dinoprostone** ($PGF_2\alpha$) [see 📖 p. 473 box].

12. **A.** True [see 📖 Table 22.1].

B. True [see 📖 p. 466].

C. False; **clomiphene** binds to oestrogen receptors in the hypothalamus and anterior pituitary [see 📖 Fig. 22.6].

D. True [see 📖 pp. 460–461].

E. False on both counts. **Anabolic steroids** (e.g. nandrolone) carry the risk of serious side effects and experts consider that it is doubtful whether they really increase athletic performance [see 📖 pp. 464–465].

F. False; **gonadorelin** needs to be given in pulsatile fashion to stimulate gonadotrophin release [see 📖 p. 466, Fig 22.6].

G. This sounds unlikely but it is true. Postmenopausal women have no ovarian oestrogen secretion or progesterone secretion, therefore no negative-feedback effect on gonadotrophin secretion. The preparation is **menotrophin** [see 📖 p. 467].

H. False; a β_2-adrenoceptor stimulant, e.g. **terbutaline**, can be used [see 📖 p. 470].

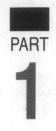

I. True [see 📖 p. 473 box].

J. True; e.g. topical gemeprost [see 📖 p. 473].

K. True [see 📖 p. 458].

L. False; it does inhibit 5α-reductase, but this enzyme converts testosterone to dihydrotestosterone.

M. True [see 📖 p. 465].

23

The haemopoietic system

BACKGROUND INFORMATION

Normal erythropoiesis requires certain exogenous substances (e.g. iron, folic acid, vitamin B_{12}) and various endogenous substances (e.g. colony-stimulating factors, erythropoietin, intrinsic factor). The main disorders of haemopoiesis are the anaemias, and the causes are:

- deficiency of essential exogenous factors
- depression of the bone marrow (due to infections, or the toxic effects of certain drugs)
- destruction of red blood cells.

The main drugs used clinically are: iron compounds (e.g. **ferrous sulphate**), **folic acid**, vitamin B_{12} preparations (e.g. **hydroxocobalamin**), **epoietin** and some colony-stimulating factors (e.g. **filgrastrim**).

QUESTIONS

1. What is the main mechanism controlling body iron?

2. What is the main pharmacological function of iron? What is the main clinical use of **iron preparations**?

3. What preparation(s) could be used to combat the effects of excessive doses of iron salts taken by mouth and how are they given?

4. **a.** What is the physiological function of **folic acid**?

   b. What is the result of folic acid deficiency?

5. In what circumstances is **epoietin** useful as a drug and why?

6. What **iron preparations** can be given parenterally? Which parenteral route is used?

7. If a laboratory report on a patient who had suffered chronic blood loss from haemorrhoids stated 'the plasma iron concentration is 2 g/100 ml', what iron preparations would you use in therapy?

8. Indicate which, if any, of the following statements are true and which false. If you think a statement is false, explain why.

   A. Ferrous iron preparations need to be converted to ferric iron for absorption.

   B. Iron is carried in the plasma bound to haemosiderin.

   C. Most of the iron which enters the plasma is derived from time-expired red blood cells.

   D. Ferritin iron is the primary storage form of iron and is in equilibrium with plasma iron.

   E. Apoferritin is a degraded form of ferritin.

   F. Intrinsic factor is essential for folic acid absorption.

   G. Intrinsic factor is secreted by gastric mucosal cells.

   H. Vitamin B$_{12}$, given orally, is essential in patients with pernicious anaemia.

   I. Vitamin B$_{12}$ is necessary for the synthesis of folate polyglutamates.

   J. Folate polyglutamate is a necessary cofactor in the synthesis of thymidylate.

   K. The transfer of iron from the carrier in the intestinal mucosal cell to either plasma transferrin or cellular ferritin depends on the iron saturation of plasma transferrin.

   L. Epoeitin is used to treat AIDS.

ANSWERS

1. The control of body iron depends on the absorptive mechanism in the intestinal mucosa, which is influenced by the body's iron stores. This has clinical significance in that excessive amounts of iron preparations taken orally or excessive iron given parenterally can cause serious adverse effects since the body has no mechanism for controlling excretion [see p. 478 box].

2. The main pharmacological function of iron is to provide material for haemoglobin synthesis, and it is only used to treat or prevent iron deficiency anaemia [see p. 478 box].

3. Some iron tablets look like sweets. Children may swallow them and acute iron toxicity can be life-threatening. **Desferrioxamine**, given parenterally, is used to chelate absorbed iron (milk might delay absorption of any iron still in the GIT) [see p. 478 box].

4. **a.** It is essential for reactions involved in DNA synthesis.

   b. Megaloblastic anaemia [see p. 483 box].

5. The anaemia of renal disease. Erythropoietin is normally produced by the kidneys and diseased kidneys produce less of it [see p. 485].

6. **Iron-dextran** or **iron-sorbitol**, usually given i.m. [see p. 479].

7. None we hope, but you would need to tell the patient to keep well away from magnets; the *total* plasma iron is **4 mg** [see Fig. 23.3]. (Note that the laboratory investigation on a patient who has suffered chronic blood loss would include measurements of total red cell count, haemoglobin values, histological study of the blood cells, etc., but would not really include plasma iron values.)

8. **A.** False; iron needs to be converted to the ferrous form to be absorbed [see p. 478 box].

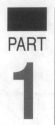
B. False; iron is carried in plasma bound to a β-globulin, transferrin. Haemosiderin is a degraded form of ferritin found intracellularly [see 📖 p. 478 box].

C. True [see 📖 p. 477].

D. True [see 📖 pp. 477–478].

E. False; apoferritin is a protein which takes up ferrous iron, oxidises it and deposits the ferric iron in its core, the complex constituting the storage form of iron, ferritin [see 📖 pp. 477–478].

F. False; it is required for **vitamin B$_{12}$** absorption [see 📖 p. 481].

G. True [see 📖 p. 481].

H. False; most deficiencies of vitamin B$_{12}$, including pernicious anaemia, are due to malabsorption of the vitamin. In the case of pernicious anaemia this is due to lack of intrinsic factor. A **vitamin B$_{12}$** preparation must be given parenterally [see 📖 pp. 483–484].

I. True [see 📖 Fig. 23.8].

J. True [see 📖 p. 483 box and Figs 23.4–23.7].

K. True [see 📖 Fig. 23.2].

L. False; it is not used to treat AIDS as such; it may be useful in the treatment of the anaemia of AIDS. For its main use see Answer 5 above.

24

Chemical transmission in the central nervous system

BACKGROUND INFORMATION

Drugs acting on the CNS have great clinical importance. The principles of chemical transmission in the CNS are the same as those in the peripheral nervous system. The complexity of the former is, however, far greater. In addition to the fact that there are multiple transmitters in CNS neurons, and multiple receptors for them to work on, the extensive interconnection and integrative functions of the CNS make evaluation difficult. The number and range of effects of neurotransmitters are steadily increasing.

QUESTIONS

1. Name the main excitatory transmitters in the CNS.

2. Name the main inhibitory transmitters in the CNS.

3. Name the monoamine transmitters. Can they be categorised as inhibitory or excitatory?

4. **Noradrenaline**

   a. What are the four receptor types for noradrenaline?

   b. What is different about some of the α_2-receptors in the CNS compared to those in the peripheral nervous system?

   c. Give three important functional roles of noradrenaline in the brain.

   d. Name an important nucleus in the brain, containing noradrenaline neurons.

5. **Dopamine**

   a. What are the main steps in the synthesis of dopamine?

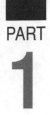

b. How many receptors are there for dopamine?

c. Which is the presynaptic dopamine receptor and what is it linked to?

d. List three important functional roles of dopamine in the brain.

e. What is the clinical importance of dopamine in the nigrostriatal pathway?

f. Name the three other major dopamine pathways.

6. 5-Hydroxytryptamine (5-HT)

a. What is the main factor regulating 5-HT synthesis?

b. Outline six important functional roles of 5-HT in the brain.

c. Name a centrally acting 5-HT analogue used for non-medical purposes. What does it do and how does it do it?

7. Acetylcholine

a. What are the main functions ascribed to CNS cholinergic pathways and which acetylcholine receptors are involved?

b. What condition is associated with a relatively selective loss of cholinergic neurons in the basal forebrain nuclei?

c. What condition is associated with hyperactivity of cholinergic neurons in the corpus striatum?

d. What are the central actions and the clinical uses of muscarinic antagonists?

8. Excitatory amino acids (EAAS)

a. Name the two main excitatory amino acid transmitters in the CNS.

b. Name the main receptor types for these.

c. What is odd about the channel associated with the NMDA receptor?

d. What is the co-agonist at the NMDA receptor and why did this finding cause a stir?

e. Would you be surprised if someone had what appeared to be a heart attack—chest pains—after massive consumption of Dim Sum?

f. What CNS processes are the NMDA receptors involved in?

9. GABA

a. What is the precursor for GABA?

b. Name the GABA receptors. Where are they located on neurons? What are their transduction mechanisms?

c. Where do **bicuculline** and **baclofen** act?

d. How do **benzodiazepines** interact with GABA systems?

10. Glycine

a. What is the principal function of glycine in the CNS? What receptors does it act on?

b. What is the antagonist at the inhibitory glycine receptor? What is its main action?

c. In which part of the CNS has glycine been shown to be important in regulation of function and what is its effect?

11. What is the pathway for production of nitric oxide in neurons?

12. What are the five categories into which psychotropic drugs can be classified?

ANSWERS

1. The excitatory amino acids are glutamate and aspartate, with some help from noradrenaline, 5-hydroxytryptamine and some peptides.

2. GABA, glycine, dopamine and some adrenoceptor actions and some peptides (enkephalins are probably quite important).

3. Noradrenaline, dopamine and 5-hydroxytryptamine. Only dopamine has a single direction of action (inhibitory whether on D_1 or D_2-receptors). The effects of the other two will vary depending on the receptor type.

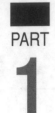

4. a. α_1, α_2, β_1, β_2, the same as in the sympathetic nervous system [see 📖 p. 495 box].

b. In the periphery, $\alpha2$ are presynaptic, whereas in the CNS many are postsynaptic as well [see 📖 p. 494].

c. It is involved in the systems controlling arousal, mood and blood pressure regulation [see 📖 p. 495 box].

d. The locus ceruleus contains a few thousand noradrenaline neurons which project to widespread areas of the brain.

5. a. Tyrosine → DOPA → dopamine, as for NA [see 📖 Fig. 7.3].

b. D_1 and D_2 are the two main receptors but both receptors can be divided into subtypes to include five receptors overall [see 📖 p. 497].

c. D_2; it is linked to adenylate cyclase, which it inhibits [see 📖 p. 499 box].

d. It is involved in the systems regulating motor control, some behavioural responses, hormone release from anterior pituitary and vomiting [see 📖 pp. 498–499].

e. This is the system that degenerates in Parkinson's disease [see 📖 p. 499 box].

f. The mesolimbic and mesocortical pathways implicated in the control of mood and emotion and the tubero-infundibular pathway from hypothalamus to pituitary involved in hormonal regulation.

6. a. The availability of tryptophan, the precursor.

b. It is involved in the systems controlling some behavioural responses, feeding behaviour, sleep/wakefulness, mood, sensory pathways (including nociception), body temperature [see 📖 p. 502 box].

c. LSD. It is a hallucinogen. It is a mixed agonist/antagonist at 5-HT receptors in the CNS [see 📖 p. 500, Ch. 32].

7. a. Arousal and learning and motor control [see 📖 p. 505 box]; nicotinic and muscarinic.

b. Dementias of the Alzheimer type (DAT) [see 📖 pp. 505 box, 524].

c. Parkinson's disease [see 📖 pp. 505 box, 527].

d. In man, **hyoscine** (used for pre-anaesthetic medication) is sedative and can cause amnesia; small doses are anti-emetic and are used to prevent travel sickness [see 📖 Fig. 19.8]. In experiments on cats, **atropine** inhibits arousal [see 📖 Fig. 24.7], but toxic doses of atropine in man cause CNS stimulation [see 📖 Ch. 6].

8. a. Glutamate and aspartate [see 📖 p. 505].

b. NMDA, AMPA, kainate, metabotropic [see 📖 Table 24.3].

c. There is a resting block by magnesium [see 📖 pp. 508–509].

d. Glycine; this transmitter was always thought to be purely inhibitory.

e. Only if the bill didn't include service. Much Chinese food contains glutamate as a 'flavour enhancer' [see 📖 p. 521].

f. In events that have been termed synaptic plasticity where changes in excitability are superimposed on normal activity. Examples include long-term potentiation (memory), epilepsy and excitotoxicity. Probably also important in spinal pain processes.

9. a. Glutamate.

b. $GABA_A$ and $GABA_B$. The former is predominantly postsynaptic whilst the latter is found presynaptically. $GABA_A$ increases Cl^- conductance, $GABA_B$ increases K^+ and decreases Ca^{2+} conductance [see 📖 Table 24.4].

c. **Bicuculline** is an antagonist at the $GABA_A$ receptor; **baclofen** is an agonist at the $GABA_B$ receptor.

d. They act at an accessory binding site on the GABA$_A$ receptor and facilitate GABA transmission [see 🔖 p. 514 box].

10. **a.** It is an inhibitory transmitter; it acts on glycine receptors which, in terms of function, resemble GABA$_A$ receptors [see 🔖 p. 514 box].

b. Strychnine. It is a convulsant [see 🔖 p. 514 box]; also useful if lacking vowels in Scrabble.

c. The ventral horn of the spinal cord; there is evidence that it can produce inhibitory hyperpolarisation, regulating motor function [see Fig. 34 for summary chart of GABA and glutamate systems].

11. An influx of calcium into neurons can activate nitric oxide synthase (there are multiple forms of the enzyme) which then converts L-arginine to NO.

12. Anxiolytic, antipsychotic, antidepressant, psychomotor stimulants and hallucinogenic drugs with the latter two not having any clinical uses.

25

Neurodegenerative disorders

PART

1

BACKGROUND INFORMATION

CNS neurons cannot divide or regenerate so that neuronal loss will have dramatic consequences. The three common degenerative conditions are Alzheimer's disease, ischaemic brain damage and Parkinson's disease. The former two are not amenable to treatment at present but the large social toll of these disorders has lead to considerable efforts to understand the mechanisms of neuronal cell death. Excessive activation of the NMDA receptor leading to elevated intracellular calcium and subsequent lethal intracellular events appears to be a key event.

Parkinson's disease is an idiopathic disease (i.e. a disease of unknown aetiology) in which there is tremor at rest, muscle rigidity and hypokinesia, often with dementia. The term 'parkinsonism' is used to describe an identical syndrome which can occur as a result of encephalitis, stroke or treatment with neuroleptic drugs.

Parkinson's disease is arguably the one disorder of the CNS where there is a clear loss of one transmitter, namely dopamine, and therefore therapy is designed to overcome the deficit. There is ample evidence that there is degeneration of the dopamine cells projecting from the substantia nigra to the corpus striatum. Dopamine is inhibitory in this area so excitatory cholinergic mechanisms are left unchecked—this is probably the main cause of the tremor. The loss of dopamine is probably the basis for the hypokinesia. The treatment is levodopa, the precursor of dopamine, coupled with adjuncts which act to limit side effects by preventing the actions of dopamine outside the CNS. Direct dopamine receptor agonists and muscarinic antagonists can also be of use.

Important drugs: levodopa, carbidopa, selegiline, domperidone, bromocriptine, benztropine.

85

Huntington's chorea

This is a hereditary disorder where a loss of GABA neurons in the corpus striatum unleashes dopamine, so causing a disorder which is the mirror image of Parkinson's disease. There is no really effective drug treatment, but neuroleptic drugs [Ch. 26] sometimes help.

QUESTIONS

1. What are the main mechanisms of excitotoxicity?

2. Why is the NMDA receptor of interest to those seeking an understanding of the basis for neuronal death?

3. What are the other names for Alzheimer's disease and ischaemic brain damage?

4. Describe the pathological features of Alzheimer's disease.

5. Why is **levodopa** used as therapy for parkinsonism rather than dopamine itself?

6. Why is **carbidopa** given with levodopa?

7. Why is **selegiline** given with levodopa? Would **clorgyline** be effective?

8. There are five main side effects of **levodopa**; two develop slowly with time, and three are acute. List these side effects.

9. What is the reason for the use of the following in Parkinson's disease:

   a. **bromocriptine**

   b. **amantidine**

   c. **benztropine**?

10. Indicate whether the statements given below are true or false. If you think a statement is false, explain why.

    A. **NMDA antagonists** may be helpful in stroke.

    B. **Levodopa**, used effectively, can control Parkinson's disease throughout a patient's life.

CHAPTER 25

C. **Levodopa** is the treatment of choice for parkinsonism or conditions like parkinsonism, however caused.

D. If **carbidopa** is used in conjunction with **levodopa** in treatment of idiopathic Parkinson's disease, much lower doses of levodopa will be effective.

E. The schizophrenia-like syndrome which can occur transiently in patients when first treated with **levodopa** is due to the increased dopamine levels in the brain.

ANSWERS

1. A maintained rise in intracellular calcium (overload) leading to an activation of proteases, free radical production, lipid peroxidation and the production of nitric oxide and arachidonic acid.

2. The NMDA receptor–channel complex when activated causes huge calcium fluxes into neurons which can lead to the events described above. Antagonists at this receptor have great potential from animal studies but as yet their clinical usefulness remains unknown.

3. 'Senile dementia' and 'stroke', respectively.

4. A loss of forebrain cholinergic neurones accompanied by amyloid plaques and neurofibrillary tangles.

5. **Levodopa** crosses the blood–brain barrier, dopamine does not.

6. **Carbidopa** inhibits dopa decarboxylase and so prevents the production of dopamine from **levodopa.** This would be counterproductive if not for the fact that carbidopa does not penetrate the brain. Thus peripheral production of dopamine and subsequent formation of noradrenaline is prevented. The peripheral side effects are reduced and more levodopa is available for conversion to dopamine in the brain, so lower doses of levodopa can be used [see 📖 p. 529 box].

7. Selegiline is a monoamine oxidase (MAO-B) inhibitor and so reduces metabolism of dopamine. **Clorgyline** is a selective MAO-A inhibitor and would not be effective because dopamine is a substrate only for MAO-B enzymes, which predominate in dopamine-containing areas in the CNS [see 🖉 p. 529, Table 29.4].

8. Slowly developing: involuntary writhing movements and 'on–off' effects. Acute: nausea, hypotension, schizophrenia-like symptoms; these may disappear after a few weeks of therapy [see 🖉 pp. 528–529].

9. a. Bromocriptine is a directly acting dopamine agonist and mimics the action of the missing dopamine.

b. Amantidine may increase dopamine release.

c. Benztropine is a muscarinic antagonist used to reduce the increased cholinergic activity responsible for the tremor.

[See 🖉 p. 530 box.]

10. A. True in theory, but the clinical benefits are, as yet, unknown.

B. False; effectiveness declines, probably due to progression of the disease [see 🖉 p. 528].

C. False; **levodopa** is the drug of choice for idiopathic Parkinson's disease but is less effective in post-encephalitic parkinsonism and is best avoided in the parkinsonism-like condition induced by neuroleptic drugs.

D. True [see 🖉 p. 530 box].

E. True [see 🖉 pp. 528–529].

26
General anaesthetic agents

BACKGROUND INFORMATION

General anaesthetics are the drugs which make surgical procedures feasible. They are given systemically, produce loss of consciousness, loss of all modalities of sensation, inhibition of many reflexes, and relaxation of skeletal muscle. Most are given either by inhalation or by the intravenous route. There are unlikely to be classic receptor-mediated events in the actions of most general anaesthetics (exceptions are the benzodiazepines and ketamine), but liposolubility is well correlated with anaesthetic potency, suggesting that interaction with the lipid membrane bilayer and/or binding to hydrophobic zones on proteins may be the basis of anaesthetic action. Anaesthetics with low blood:gas partition coefficients cause rapid induction and recovery and those with high liposolubility may accumulate in fat.

Important anaesthetics:
Given by inhalation: **ether, halothane, nitrous oxide, enflurane**.
Given by injection: **thiopentone, etomidate, ketamine, propofol**. These are generally used for induction.

QUESTIONS

1. a. What is the relation between liposolubility and potency of an anaesthetic?

b. What is MAC?

c. What is meant by the blood:gas partition coefficient of an anaesthetic?

2. What determines **a.** the speed of induction and **b.** recovery, with inhalation anaesthetics?

3. Which is more susceptible to the action of general anaesthetics: synaptic transmission or axonal conduction?

4. What are the main neurophysiological changes produced by general anaesthetics?

5. Which two areas in the brain are thought to be associated with the unconsciousness produced by general anaesthetics?

6. Give an example of a drug which would be used to elicit the following phenomena, listing one drug for each: **a.** rapid induction; **b.** maintenance of anaesthesia; **c.** analgesia; **d.** muscle paralysis.

7. What is the main mechanism by which the action of inhalational anaesthetics is terminated?

8. What are the general advantages and disadvantages of intravenous anaesthetics?

9. Indicate whether the following statements are true or false. If you think a statement is false, explain why.

   A. An anaesthetic with a high blood:gas partition coefficient will cause rapid induction.

   B. Nitrous oxide has a low solubility in blood and lipid.

   C. Metabolism of anaesthetics is important in terminating their actions.

   D. Metabolism of anaesthetics is important in toxicity.

   E. Halothane is an example of an anaesthetic which is not metabolised.

   F. Ether is a widely used anaesthetic because it is non-explosive.

   G. Halothane has a reasonable speed of induction and recovery but can cause a reduction in blood pressure.

   H. Nitrous oxide produces analgesia during stage 1 anaesthesia.

I. Intravenous anaesthetics produce a slower induction than inhalational anaesthetics.

J. Thiopentone is a barbiturate.

K. Thiopentone is highly liposoluble and enters the brain rapidly.

L. Thiopentone accumulates in fat and so is useful as a maintenance anaesthetic.

M. Diazepam and **ketamine** are used as maintenance anaesthetics.

N. Diazepam produces a state of dissociative anaesthesia.

O. Tubocurarine is used during operations with general anaesthetics as an analgesic.

10. Figure 16 shows data for the equilibration of various general anaesthetic agents in man.

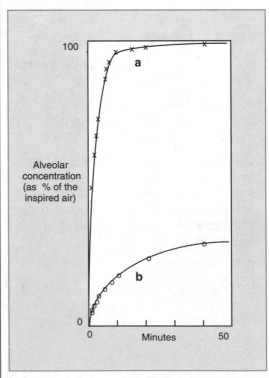

Fig. 16 The rate of equilibration of two inhalation anaesthetics in man. The curves show alveolar concentration which closely reflects arterial blood concentration.

a. Which curve gives the data for **nitrous oxide** and which for **ether**?

b. Which characteristic(s) of the two agents result in the difference in equilibration?

ANSWERS

1. a. Linear; the more liposoluble the more potent the anaesthetic will be [see 📖 Fig. 26.1].

b. MAC is minimum alveolar concentration, a measure of the amount of anaesthetic needed to prevent a response to a standard painful stimulus in 50% of patients tested [see 📖 p. 533, Fig. 26.1].

c. Roughly, if the anaesthetic is allowed to distribute itself between equal volumes of blood and air under standard conditions, the partition coefficient is the ratio of the amount in blood to the amount in air at equilibrium. For **halothane**, for example, this ratio is 2.4:1 [see 📖 Table 26.1]. This property of an anaesthetic is a main factor in determining the rate of induction of anaesthesia and subsequent recovery [see 📖 p. 538].

2. Both are determined primarily by the solubility of the agent in blood (blood:gas partition coefficient) and its solubility in lipid (oil solubility) [see 📖 Table 26.1, Fig. 26.3, p. 540 box].

3. The former [see 📖 p. 540 box].

4. Unconsciousness, loss of response to painful stimuli, loss of motor reflexes [see 📖 p. 540 box].

5. The reticular activating system and the hippocampus [see 📖 p. 537 box].

6. a. Thiopentone (or other intravenous anaesthetics) or nitrous oxide [see 📖 p. 546 box, Table 26.1].

b. Halothane (or other inhalation anaesthetics) [see 📖 p. 543 box].

c. Morphine (or other opiod analgesics) [see 📖 Ch. 31].

d. Tubocurarine (or other neuro-muscular blockers) [see 📖 p. 139 box].

7. They are exhaled. Some are partly metabolised but this does not influence their duration of action [see 📖 p. 540 box].

8. Intravenous anaesthetics (**thiopentone**, **etomidate**, **ketamine**, **propofol**) act very rapidly—more rapidly even than the fastest acting inhalation agents. They are therefore very useful for induction. They have the added advantage that an injection doesn't have the quality of menace which a mask over the face can have to an apprehensive patient. They are unsatisfactory for maintenance of anaesthesia because, unlike inhalation agents, there is no moment-to-moment control of anaesthesia. With an inhalation agent, when you remove the mask or cease giving the anaesthetic, elimination commences immediately; with an intravenous agent, once the drug is in, it's in, and you have to wait for it to be metabolised and/or excreted before the blood level drops. Some intravenous anaesthetics can be used as sole agents, however, for very short surgical procedures, e.g. draining a rectal abscess, setting a fracture, etc.

9. A. False; the opposite is true [see 📖 Table 26.1].

B. True; its blood:gas partition coefficient is 0.47:1 (as compared with 12:1 for ether); this is the basis for the rapid induction and recovery with nitrous oxide and the slow induction and recovery with ether. Its oil:gas partition coefficient is 1.4:1 (as compared with 65:1 for ether); this determines its potency [see 📖 Fig. 26.1].

C. False as explained in Answer 7 above [but see D below].

D. True [see 📖 p. 617].

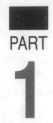

E. No, 30% is metabolised [see 🖋 p. 540].

F. False; it is little used these days. In addition to being explosive it is irritant, and both induction and recovery are prolonged [see 🖋 p. 543 box, Table 26.1].

G. True [see 🖋 p. 543 box].

H. True; hence it is used during childbirth and at the scene of an accident [see 🖋 p. 542].

I. False; the opposite is true, hence the use of **thiopentone** to induce anaesthesia [see Answer 8 above].

J. True [see 🖋 p. 544].

K. True [see 🖋 p. 544].

L. False; it would certainly accumulate if, after the dose used for induction, repeated doses were given for maintenance, but the duration and depth of anaesthesia would increase with each dose and could reach danger level. The accumulation in fat, with later release, would produce a long 'hangover' effect [see 🖋 pp. 544–545, Fig. 26.7].

M. True [see 🖋 p. 544].

N. False; ketamine does this, by acting as a channel blocker at the NMDA receptor [see 🖋 p. 546 box].

O. False; **tubocurarine** is a non-depolarising neuromuscular-blocking agent used to paralyse the muscles. **Opiates** are used for their analgesic effects; their use during surgical operations allows surgical procedures to be carried out at lower levels of general anaesthetic than would otherwise be required.

10. a. Nitrous oxide is curve **a**; **ether** is curve **b**.

b. Mainly their respective blood:gas partition coefficients; the *lower* the solubility in blood, the faster the process of equilibration [see Answer 9 above and 🖋 pp. 538–540].

27

Anxiolytic and hypnotic drugs

BACKGROUND INFORMATION

Anxiety and sleep disorders are among the most widely encountered problems in clinical practice, and the benzodiazepine drugs, relatively safe for the treatment of both of these disorders, account for a large proportion of prescriptions in the western world. Beta blockers and some agents acting on the 5-HT transmitter system are also used to treat anxiety. The benzodiazepines produce their effects by actions on GABA systems which in turn may well act on 5-HT downstream. In addition to the above effects, the benzodiazepines are centrally acting muscle relaxants and anticonvulsants; some short-acting ones are used in anaesthesia regimes for surgery because of their hypnotic, anxiolytic and amnesic effects. The previous use of the barbiturates has declined because of their low safety margin.

Drugs used clinically include: benzodiazepines (e.g. **diazepam**, **nitrazepam**), benzodiazepine antagonists (e.g. **flumazenil**), 5-HT receptor agonists (e.g. **buspirone**), barbiturates (e.g. **pentobarbitone**).

A summary chart of benzodiazepine and barbiturate action is included in Part 2, Figure 34.

QUESTIONS

1. Define: **a.** anxiolytic; **b.** hypnotic.

2. List the four main classes of drugs used to treat **a.** anxiety and **b.** insomnia, stating which is used for which.

3. List the four main actions of the benzodiazepines.

4. What are the effects of the benzodiazepines on REM sleep and slow wave (SW) sleep?

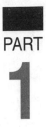

5. In treating anxiety, can sedation be avoided?

6. Are all the benzodiazepines anticonvulsant?

7. Where are the binding sites for benzodiazepines?

8. What happens to chloride channels when benzodiazepines bind to their sites?

9. What are inverse agonists?

10. Are benzodiazepines liposoluble?

11. Why might there be problems with benzodiazepines in the elderly?

12. If the 5-HT autoreceptor is the 5-HT_{1A} subtype and 5-HT is believed to be involved in anxiety, what does this indicate about the effects of an agonist such as **buspirone** in the treatment of anxiety?

13. What are the differences in the side effects of 5-HT agonist drugs as compared with those of the benzodiazepines in the treatment of anxiety?

14. Barbiturates open chloride channels independently of GABA function. Would they then be safer than benzodiazepines?

15. Are barbiturates important in interactions with other drugs and, if so, how?

16. Give examples of benzodiazepines with the following characteristics:

   a. short-acting, used as a hypnotic (give $t_{1/2}$)

   b. long-acting, used as an anti-convulsant (give $t_{1/2}$)

   c. short $t_{1/2}$ of parent compound, long $t_{1/2}$ of active metabolite.

17. What effects are likely to occur in an individual who takes 20 times the prescribed dose of **a.** nitrazepam or **b.** pentobarbitone? Is there a pharmacological solution to the problem(s) which would result?

18. Indicate whether the following statements are true or false. If you think a statement is false, explain why.

   A. Benzodiazepines bind to a site on the $GABA_B$ receptor.

   B. Benzodiazepine use can lead to tolerance which is due to markedly increased activity of the hepatic drug-metabolising enzymes.

   C. Unlike barbiturates, benzodiazepines such as **nitrazepam** do not cause day-after impairment of tasks requiring good hand–eye coordination.

   D. The binding of benzodiazepines to postsynaptic sites results in facilitation of opening of Cl^- channels by the relevant transmitter, with resultant depolarisation.

   E. **Diazepam** is converted, in part, to **temazepam** in the body.

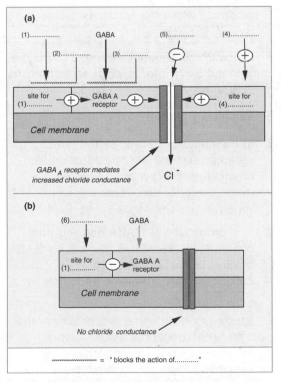

Fig. 17 Schematic diagram of the interactions at the GABA receptor and the chloride channel. The drugs or drug groups that act at the sites are indicated by 1, 2, 3, 4, 5, 6 in (a) and (b). Note that drug (6) in (b) decreases the affinity of GABA for the $GABA_A$ receptor.

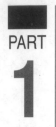

19. Figure 17 is a schematic diagram of the interactions at the GABA receptor and the chloride channel. What drugs or drug groups act at the sites indicated by 1, 2, 3, 4, 5, 6 in **(a)** and **(b)**?

Note that drug (6) in **(b)** decreases the affinity of GABA for the $GABA_A$ receptor.

ANSWERS

1. **a.** A drug used to treat anxiety; **b.** a drug used to treat insomnia.

2. Benzodiazepines (both); 5-HT agonists (anxiety); barbiturates (both) but little used now; beta blockers (anxiety) [see 📖 p. 550 box].

3. Reduction in anxiety, increase in sleep, anticonvulsant activity and muscle relaxation [see 📖 p. 559 box].

4. REM sleep is only slightly reduced, SW sleep more so and there is a rebound insomnia when the treatment ceases [see 📖 p. 551].

5. Not with the benzodiazepines but maybe with the 5-HT agents, such as **buspirone** [see 📖 pp. 559 box, 560 box].

6. Yes [see 📖 p. 559 box].

7. In the complex formed by the $GABA_A$ receptor and the associated chloride channel on postsynaptic neuronal membranes; binding sites are found widely in the CNS [see 📖 Fig. 27.4].

8. The probability of GABA opening the channel is increased. If there is no GABA binding to the receptor, the benzodiazepines have no effect [see 📖 p. 553, Fig. 27.4].

9. Drugs (such as some β-**carbolines**) that bind to the benzodiazepine site but produce anxiety and convulsions, the opposite effects to the benzodiazepines [see 📖 pp. 555, 559 box, Fig. 27.4].

10. Yes; hence they penetrate the brain well and can be given orally.

11. In the elderly, metabolism is reduced and renal function can be impaired, so that accumulation of most benzodiazepines can occur. The glucuronide conjugation reactions are less affected by age than the oxidative reactions; so benzodiazepines which undergo conjugation but not oxidation, such as **lorazepam** [see 📖 Fig. 27.5], will be rather less likely to cumulate in the elderly.

12. Take a deep breath! **Buspirone**, by acting as an agonist on the autoreceptor, will reduce the release of 5-HT and so reduce activity in the neuronal systems believed to be implicated in anxiety. It is thought that the enhancement of GABA transmission produced by the benzodiazepines in turn acts to reduce 5-HT activity so the same final result is achieved by both approaches [see 📖 pp. 560 box, 559 box].

13. There is less sedation and fewer motor effects with the 5-HT agonists, and, more importantly, they do not potentiate the effects of alcohol and other CNS depressants.

14. No. There is no ceiling on their inhibitory effects (including depression of respiration), so overdose can be fatal.

15. Barbiturates induce hepatic metabolising enzymes and so will increase the metabolism of many other drugs. This is an example of an important drug interaction [see 📖 p. 560, Table 42.2].

16. **a.** temazepam, $t_{1/2}$ 8 h; **b.** clonazepam, $t_{1/2}$ 50 h; **c.** flurazepam, $t_{1/2}$ 1 h, $t_{1/2}$ of active metabolite 40–200 h [see 📖 Table 27.1].

17. **a.** **Nitrazepam** overdosage causes deep, prolonged sleep, without depression of respiration or cardiovascular function; **flumazenil** could be an effective antagonist, but it is very short-acting and would need to be given by infusion [see 📖 p. 557].

b. **Pentobarbitone** in overdosage depresses respiration and cardiovascular function, and 20 times the normal hypnotic dose is likely to be fatal. There is no pharmacological antagonist. Therapy of overdosage involves the use of respirators, dialysis, etc. Between 1959 and 1974 (before benzodiazepines were generally available) there were 27 000 deaths from self-administered barbiturate overdosage.

18. **A.** False; $GABA_A$ not $GABA_B$ [see 🖉 p. 559 box].

B. False; benzodiazepines do produce some degree of tolerance, but this is mainly tissue tolerance. They have only minimal effects on the hepatic microsomal enzymes [see 🖉 p. 558].

C. False; the long-acting benzodiazepines, of which **nitrazepam** is one ($t_{1/2}$ 28 h), do cause day-after impairment of tasks requiring good hand–eye coordination; they also cause some drowsiness. Shorter-acting benzodiazepines, such as **temazepam** are less likely to have these effects [see 🖉 pp. 557–558, Table 27.1].

D. False; hyperpolarisation and consequent neuronal inhibition result from the opening of the Cl⁻ channel [see 🖉 p. 553].

E. True [see 🖉 Fig. 27.5].

19. **(a)** (1) **Benzodiazepines** [see 🖉 Fig. 27.4]; the benzodiazepine-binding site on the $GABA_A$ receptor exists in two forms; the one depicted here, when occupied by a benzodiazepine, facilitates GABA binding and thus the effect of GABA on chloride conductance.

(2) **Flumazenil** is an antagonist at the benzodiazepine site on the $GABA_A$ receptor [see 🖉 p. 559].

(3) **Bicuculline** is an antagonist of GABA at the $GABA_A$ receptor [see 🖉 Table 24.4, p. 514 box].

(4) **Barbiturates** potentiate the effect of GABA on the $GABA_A$ receptor by binding to a site separate from the benzodiazepines [see 🖉 p. 560].

(5) **Picrotoxin** blocks the chloride channel associated with the $GABA_A$ receptor [see 🖉 p. 514 box].

(b) (6) Inverse agonists (e.g. β-**carbolines**) bind selectively to the benzodiazepine-binding site on the $GABA_A$ receptor when it is in the conformation which decreases affinity for GABA; they thus block the effect of GABA on chloride conductance, i.e. the chloride channel remains closed [see 🖉 p. 555, Fig. 27.4].

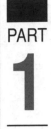

PART

1

28

Neuroleptic drugs

BACKGROUND

The terms 'neuroleptic', 'antipsychotic drug', 'antischizophrenic drug' and 'major tranquilliser' are used interchangeably. All the agents currently used are antagonists of dopamine. Nevertheless, there are only a few studies showing that dopamine function is elevated in schizophrenia, so the primary deficit may be elsewhere. There are three main classes of 'typical' neuroleptics: the phenothiazines, the butyrophenones and the thioxanthines. Several other agents are classed as 'atypical' neuroleptics. They all have the same primary pharmacological profile of being dopamine antagonists although they have varying actions on other transmitter systems. Because of their ability to reduce dopamine function they are also antiemetics, can cause Parkinson-like symptoms and reduce the secretion of prolactin. Tardive dyskinesia can develop slowly during treatment, as the term suggests; it is difficult to reverse.

Main drugs: chlorpromazine, haloperidol and **flupenthixol** (an example of each of the three classes above respectively). An atypical neuroleptic is **clozapine**.

QUESTIONS

1. Name three important types of psychosis.

2. What are the four main symptoms of schizophrenia? Clues:

    a. I know all the pharmacology there is to know, but they won't believe me.

    b. St Xavier of Santiago will tell me the answers in the exam.

    c. I knew lots of pharmacology until the CIA extracted all I knew about adrenoceptors.

    d. I'm not sitting next to *him* in the exam.

3. Are the positive or the negative symptoms of schizophrenia more amenable to treatment?

4. How many types of **dopamine** receptors are there believed to be and which one is seemingly the most important in the effects of neuroleptics?

5. What would a plot of potency of dopamine D_2 antagonism against therapeutic effectiveness look like for a series of neuroleptics?

6. In general the neuroleptics have actions on four other transmitter systems. What are they and are these effects relevant to the therapeutic profile of these drugs?

7. What is the relationship between neuroleptics and vomiting? What is the basis of the relationship?

8. What is tardive dyskinesia?

9. List five main side effects of the neuroleptics.

10. How often and by what route are the neuroleptics given?

11. Indicate whether the following statements are true or false. If you think a statement is false, explain why.

    A. All neuroleptic drugs are agonists at D_2 receptors.

    B. Sulpiride, an 'atypical' neuroleptic, has fairly selective effects on dopamine D_2-receptors as compared with **chlorpromazine** or **haloperidol**.

    C. Clozapine has many extrapyramidal effects.

    D. Neuroleptic drugs increase **prolactin** secretion by stimulating D_2-receptors in the anterior pituitary.

    E. The response to neuroleptics takes days or weeks to develop, which suggests that the action of these drugs is related to the increase in dopamine D_1-receptors in limbic structures.

F. The two main types of motor disorder which can occur as side effects of many neuroleptic drugs—parkinsonism and tardive dyskinesia—are reversible and will decline as treatment progresses.

ANSWERS

1. Important psychoses are schizophrenia and the affective disorders (depression and anxiety, mania)—which are not necessarily associated with any obvious disease or damage to the brain—and organic psychoses which are caused by CNS injury or disease [see 📖 p. 562].

2. **a.** Delusions (often paranoid).

   b. Hallucinations, hearing voices, etc.

   c. Thought disorders (particularly the idea that thoughts are interfered with by outside agencies).

   d. Withdrawal from social contacts.

   [See 📖 p. 562.]

3. The positive symptoms seem to respond better (the first three in the answer to Question 2), possibly because the negative symptoms, the withdrawing from social contacts and the blunting of emotions, result from organic changes (e.g. atrophy of the brain) [see 📖 p. 562].

4. Five. The D_1 and the D_2 seem to be the major types, with the D_5-receptor being related to the former and the D_3 and D_4 being subtypes of the D_2-receptor. The D_2 is the more important therapeutic target but drugs acting on D_4-receptors such as clozapine may have fewer extrapyramidal side effects than the others and have been claimed to have effectiveness against the negative symptoms [see 📖 p. 568 box].

5. A linear positive relationship, showing that there is a clear correlation between

affinity for dopamine D_2-receptors and clinical potency [see 📖 Fig. 28.1].

6. Many have antimuscarinic, adrenoceptor blocking and antihistamine actions. The consequences are thought to be, respectively: fewer extrapyramidal effects, orthostatic hypotension and sedation. In addition, the thioxanthines and atypical drugs have 5-HT_2-receptor blocking effects although the consequences are unclear [see 📖 p. 654, Table 26.1].

7. Neuroleptics have anti-emetic action. **Dopamine** is a transmitter in the chemoreceptor trigger zone of the brain stem and neuroleptics are dopamine antagonists [see 📖 pp. 569–570, Fig. 19.8].

8. Involuntary movements, late in onset. This resembles the dyskinesia which occurs after long-continued levodopa therapy in patients with Parkinson's disease [see 📖 pp. 572, 530 box].

9. Extrapyramidal disturbances, increased prolactin release, sedation, dry mouth, blurred vision and hypotension. Some may cause neutropenia [see 📖 p. 572 box].

10. Orally or i.m. once or twice a day; or i.m. in the form of depot injections (slow-release) every 2–4 months.

11. **A.** False; they are antagonists at D_2-receptors [see 📖 p. 568 box].

    B. True; in common with **pimozide**, it has little or no effect on dopamine D_1, H_1, 5-HT, α-adrenoceptor or muscarinic receptors [see 📖 Table 28.1].

    C. False; **clozapine** has few extrapyramidal effects, and the same is true of **thioridazine** (a phenothiazine). However, some phenothiazines (namely **fluophenazine** and **trifluperazine**) have marked extrapyramidal effects, as do the butyrophenones (**haloperidol**, **droperidol**) [see 📖 Table 28.1].

    D. False; most (but not all) neuroleptic drugs increase prolactin secretion, but

they do so by antagonising the inhibitory action of dopamine on prolactin release which is mediated through D_2-receptors in the anterior pituitary [see p. 571].

E. False; since many neuroleptics have little or no effect on D_1-receptors, but the statement may be true for D_2-receptors [see p. 568 box].

F. False; the parkinsonism-like symptoms can develop quite rapidly and often decline as treatment progresses; but the tardive dyskinesia (which occurs in 10% of neuroleptic-treated patients) develops late and is often irreversible [see p. 570].

29

Drugs used in affective disorders

BACKGROUND INFORMATION

The affective disorders, mania and depression, are disturbances of mood, unlike the alterations in thought processes that typify schizophrenia. The monoamine theory of depression holds that this disorder results from a functional deficit in the monoamine transmitters, principally noradrenaline (NA) but also 5-HT. Although there are problems with this theory, most (though not all) treatment regimes are based on manipulation of these two transmitter systems.

Drugs used clinically include: tricyclic antidepressants (TCAs) (**amitriptyline, imipramine**), monoamine oxidase inhibitors (MAOIs) (e.g. **phenelzine, tranylcypromine**), selective uptake blockers of 5-HT (e.g. **fluoxetine**), 'atypical' antidepressants (e.g. **iprindole, mianserin**), **lithium**.

QUESTIONS

1. What is the main mechanism of action of:

   a. the **tricyclic antidepressants** (TCAs)?

   b. the **monoamine oxidase inhibitors** (MAOIs)?

2. If the following drugs were to be used in depressed patients, what would be the effect on mood: up, down or no effect? What is the basis for the effect, if any?

   a. tricyclic antidepressants

   b. monoamine oxidase inhibitors

   c. methyldopa

   d. methyltyrosine.

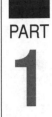

3. What are the three pieces of evidence that undermine the idea that antidepressants simply increase noradrenergic transmission in the CNS?

4. Indicate whether the following statements are true or false. If you think a statement is false, explain why.

    a. TCAs:

        A. include the drugs, **imipramine** and **amitriptyline**.

        B. block the re-uptake of noradrenaline and **5-HT**.

        C. are all metabolised to inactive forms.

        D. often have α_2-adrenoceptor blocking effects.

        E. cause diarrhoea and increased blood pressure as side effects.

        F. are safe even with an overdose.

    b. MAOIs:

        A. all act on both forms of MAO, A and B.

        B. effect on MAO-A, rather than MAO-B, is probably more important for antidepressant action.

        C. cause an increase in noradrenaline only within the cytoplasm of the nerve terminal.

        D. commonly cause hypotension as a side effect.

        E. can cause CNS stimulation and arousal.

        F. should not be used in conjunction with a Camembert and Marmite sandwich.

        G. cause a rapid increase in the brain content of 5-HT, NA, dopamine.

    c. **A.** 'Atypical' antidepressants, unlike MAOIs, have a rapid onset of action.

        B. Fluoxetine and **maprotiline** are selective NA uptake blockers.

        C. Mianserin and **trazodone** have distinct sedative properties.

        D. Nomifensine tends to cause behavioural stimulation and may interfere with sleep.

        E. Most atypical antidepressants interact with the opiate **pethidine**, causing high fever and hypotension.

        F. Mianserin may affect the bone marrow and thus repeated blood counts should be carried out.

        G. Atypical antidepressants may safely be combined with MAOI.

5. What are the advantages of the selective 5-HT uptake inhibitors as compared with the tricyclic antidepressants?

6. **a.** Name an antidepressant which has a *selective* effect on noradrenaline uptake.

    b. Name an antidepressant which has a *selective* effect on 5-HT uptake.

    c. Name an antidepressant which has *equal* effects on both 5-HT and noradrenaline uptake.

7. Is there evidence for ECT being effective?

8. **a.** What is **lithium** used for?

    b. What are the two main intracellular actions of lithium?

ANSWERS

1. **a.** TCAs act on monoaminergic nerve terminals, inhibiting noradrenaline and 5-HT uptake.

    b. MAOIs inhibit monoamine oxidase in the brain; the breakdown of noradrenaline and 5-HT is decreased and intracellular stores of these transmitters increase.

2. **a.** Up; due to increased action of NA and/or 5-HT through block of re-uptake [see 🖉 p. 583 box, Table 29.3].

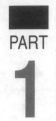

b. Up; due to increased intracellular NA and 5-HT through block of breakdown [see 📖 p. 583 box, Table 29.4].

c. Down; false transmitter, NA reduced [see 📖 Table 8.5] (used as antihypertensive in some patients, not used to treat depression).

d. Down; inhibits NA synthesis [see 📖 Table 7.4] (occasionally used to treat phaeochromocytoma, not used to treat depression).

[See 📖 Table 29.1.]

3. (i) The lag between administration and therapeutic benefit (weeks) is much longer than the biochemical effects of the drugs (hours).

(ii) The atypical antidepressants are effective but do not all have obvious effects on monoamine function (which is why they are termed 'atypical') [see 📖 p. 577, Table 29.5].

(iii) The fact that drugs acting on 5-HT systems are as effective if not more effective.

4. **a. A.** True [see 📖 p. 580].

B. True; but selectivity for NA or 5-HT can vary between the parent compound and its metabolites [see 📖 Table 29.3].

C. False; many are converted to active metabolites [see 📖 p. 586 box].

D. True [see 📖 p. 584].

E. False; exactly the opposite [see 📖 p. 673 box].

F. False [see 📖 p. 586 box].

b. A. False; **selegiline** is selective for type B and **clorgyline** for type A [see 📖 Table 29.4]. But note that selegiline is not used for depression.

B. True [see A above and 📖 p. 587].

C. False; the terminal leaks noradrenaline as a result of increased NA which is consequent on

the decrease in breakdown; MAO inhibitors will increase the response of agents (**amphetamine**, **tyramine** in cheese, etc) which displace NA from vesicle to cytoplasm because they increase the pool of NA which can leak out [see 📖 pp. 587–588].

D. True; this may occur in spite of the fact that increased NA release by indirect sympathomimetics also occurs [see 📖 p. 589].

E. True [see 📖 p. 589 box].

F. True; these substances contain tyramine [see 📖 p. 589 box].

G. True [see 📖 p. 588].

c. A. False; the delay in clinical response is similar to that seen with both MAO inhibitors and the tricyclic antidepressants [see 📖 p. 592 box].

B. False; **maprotiline** selectively blocks NA uptake, but **fluoxetine** is a specific 5-HT uptake blocker [see 📖 Table 27.5].

C. True [see 📖 Table 29.5].

D. True [see 📖 Table 29.5].

E. False; this statement is true for interaction of **pethidine** with MAOIs [see 📖 p. 589 box].

F. True.

G. False; because of the mechanism of action of the two groups of drugs, serious interactions could occur. There should be at least a fortnight between the use of MAOIs and agents which block amine uptake.

5. The selective 5-HT uptake blockers have no anticholinergic and cardiovascular effects, low acute toxicity, and lack the food reactions seen with MAOIs. However, aggression and cardiovascular collapse are disadvantages as is their high price. Examples include **fluoxetine** and **paroxetine**.

6. **a.** You could have chosen from **maprotiline**, **nomifensine**.

b. You could have chosen from **paroxetine**, **fluoxetine**.

c. Amitriptyline (**nortriptyline** would not have been far out).

[See ✎ Fig 29.4.]

7. Yes, especially in unipolar depressive states [see ✎ p. 592].

8. **a.** Mania [see ✎ p. 594 box].

b. A reduction in hormonal stimulated cyclic AMP production and an inhibition of InsP$_3$ formation [see ✎ p. 594 box].

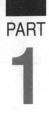

30
Antiepileptic drugs and centrally acting muscle relaxants

PART

1

BACKGROUND INFORMATION

Two types of motor disorders are dealt with here—epilepsy and muscle spasm.

Epilepsy

Epilepsy is characterised by seizures produced by abnormal discharges of groups of neurons. The seizures can be partial or generalised depending on the size of the area of brain involved. Generalised seizures can be tonic–clonic seizures (grand mal, which is accompanied by a loss of consciousness) or absence seizures (petit mal). Partial seizures include Jacksonian epilepsy and psychomotor epilepsy. Some partial seizures may become generalised.

The neurochemical basis of epilepsy is not at all clear. It may be associated with enhanced excitatory amino acid transmission, impaired inhibitory transmission or abnormal electrical properties of the relevant neurons. The content of the fast excitatory transmitter, glutamate, is often found to be raised in areas surrounding an epileptic focus. Therapy is aimed at reducing excitation or increasing inhibition.

Important drugs: phenytoin, carbamazepine, sodium valproate, benzodiazepines. A summary chart which includes several antiepileptic drugs (Fig. 34) is included in Part 2 [see also Fig. 17].

Muscle spasm

There can be an increase in skeletal muscle tone following either: (i) local injury or birth injury or (ii) cerebral vascular disorders. These can be alleviated with either **benzodiazepines** or **baclofen**, respectively.

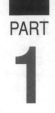

PART

1

QUESTIONS

1. What are the two main mechanisms of action of anticonvulsant drugs?

2. Why is the NMDA receptor of interest to those seeking an understanding of the basis for some forms of epilepsy?

3. Name three drugs used to treat epilepsy which have actions on GABA systems.

4. How is **phenytoin** thought to act?

5. List the main side effects of phenytoin.

6. What disorder, other than epilepsy, is **carbamazepine** used to treat?

7. What is 'status epilepticus'? How might it be treated?

8. **Ethosuximide** is used in a certain type of epilepsy. Name the type.

9. **Phenobarbitone**, like other barbiturates, acts on GABA systems. How does this interaction occur and why is it only part of the explanation for the effects of phenobarbitone?

10. What is the main side effect of both **benzodiazepines** and **barbiturates** in maintenance therapy for epilepsy?

11. Why are the pharmacokinetic aspects of the action of **phenytoin** important?

12. On what receptor(s) does **baclofen** act and which part of the CNS is important in its effects?

13. Indicate whether the statements given below are true or false. If you think a statement is false, explain why.

   A. Phenytoin is used to treat absence seizures.

   B. Phenytoin produces effects independently of sodium channel opening kinetics.

   C. Carbamazepine is a drug of choice for partial seizures and tonic–clonic seizures.

   D. Benzodiazepines enhance the effect of the inhibitory transmitter GABA.

   E. Valproate is only effective in partial seizures.

   F. Phenytoin and **carbamazepine**, given together, may result in reduced plasma concentrations of both.

   G. Phenytoin is converted to **phenobarbitone** in the body.

   H. Among the important unwanted effects which can occur with **carbamazepine** are hyperplasia, hirsutism and megaloblastic anaemia.

   I. If sedation becomes a problem with **benzodiazepines**, when these are used to treat epilepsy, the drug(s) should be stopped immediately.

   J. Vigabatrin acts by inhibiting GABA-transaminase.

   K. Lamotrigine is a GABA uptake inhibitor.

ANSWERS

1. (i) Reduction of electrical excitability of cell membranes, possibly through use-dependent block of Na^+ channels.

   (ii) Enhancement of GABA-mediated neuronal inhibition [see 📙 p. 600 box].

2. The NMDA receptor–channel complex for glutamate has characteristics which may underlie the neuronal activity in epilepsy and might also explain the cell death observed [see 📙 pp. 509, 598].

3. You could choose from **valproate**, **phenobarbitone**, **benzodiazepines** and **vigabatrin** [see Fig. 34 in Part 2 and 📙 Table 30.1].

4. By use-dependent block of Na^+ channels; it may bind inside sodium channels and block high frequency but not low frequency discharges of neurons [see Fig. 34 and 📙 Table 30.1].

5. Vertigo, headache, confusion, hyperplasia of the gums, megaloblastic anaemia, extra hair growth and

hypersensitivity reactions [see 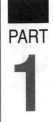 Table 30.1].

6. Trigeminal neuralgia [see 🔖 p. 603].

7. A condition where tonic–clonic seizures follow one another without the patient regaining consciousness. Urgent treatment is necessary; i.v. infusion of **cinazepam** may be used.

8. Absence seizures [see 🔖 Table 30.1].

9. Barbiturates enhance the effects of GABA, probably by acting near the associated chloride channel [see Fig. 34]. However, the degree of therapeutic efficacy does not fit well with efficacy on GABA transmission for a range of barbiturates [see 🔖 pp. 599–600].

10. Sedation [see 🔖 Table 30.1].

11. **Phenytoin** metabolism manifests zero-order kinetics (saturation kinetics), i.e. it is metabolised at a constant rate, which is independent of the plasma concentration. Thus, as the dose is increased, the plasma half-life (which is already 20 hours) also increases, and the plasma concentration varies disproportionately with the dose. There is only a small 'window' in the plasma concentration in which phenytoin is effective without causing toxic effects. Furthermore, other factors (e.g. other drugs) affect its concentration [see 🔖 Fig. 30.3, pp. 94–96].

12. GABA$_B$ receptors in the spinal cord, possibly reducing proprioceptive input.

13. **A.** False; all types of epilepsy *except* absence seizures [see 🔖 Table 30.1].

B. False; it produces a use-dependent block.

C. True [see 🔖 p. 606 box].

D. True [see 🔖 Table 30.1].

E. False; it can be used in most types and is a drug of choice in absence seizures.

F. True; they are both enzyme inducers [see 🔖 pp. 601, 604].

G. False; **primidone** is largely converted to phenobarbitone [see 🔖 Table 30.1].

H. False; these are some of the unwanted effects associated with **phenytoin** [see 🔖 Table 30.1].

I. False; abrupt withdrawal of **benzodiazepines** (or **barbiturates**) can precipitate rebound epileptic seizures. This may occur with other antiepileptic drugs.

J. True [see Fig. 34 and 🔖 Table 30.1].

K False; it is not clear how **lamotrigine** acts—it may block Na$^+$ channels.

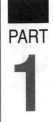

PART

1

31
Analgesic drugs

BACKGROUND INFORMATION

Pain is a subjective experience; it comprises both emotional aspects, due to the unpleasant nature of the phenomenon, and sensory aspects. The sensation initially arises from the activation of the peripheral terminals of sensory C-fibres (and to some extent Aδ-fibres) in response to mechanical and thermal stimuli. In the case of tissue damage, chemical mediators of pain such as the prostanoids, bradykinin and 5-HT activate the C-fibres and also cause vaso-dilatation which may lead to oedema. Prosta-glandins sensitise the C-fibres to the action of these mediators. At their central terminals in the spinal cord, the bipolar C-fibres release peptides (such as the tachykinin family, e.g. substance P) and also glutamate; these activate spinal cord neurons which, in turn and via ascending projections, activate supraspinal areas such as the reticular formation, thalamus and cortex. The activation of descending inhibitory pathways from the midbrain and brain stem, using the transmitters noradrenaline and 5-hydroxytryptamine, and the involvement of endogenous opioid systems, are some of the means by which the final message is processed and altered by neural systems. Three different receptors (μ, δ, and κ) are implicated in the functioning of the endogenous opioid systems. Acute pain can be distinguished from chronic pain, in which the processes leading to hyper-algesia and allodynia are becoming understood.

Analgesics are drugs which relieve pain without causing unconsciousness, and the main drugs currently used for this are the morphine-like drugs (opiates) and the non-steroidal anti-inflammatory drugs (NSAIDs). Several novel analgesics are likely to become available in the near future, including bradykinin antagonists, drugs affecting the monoamines and alternatives to morphine. Morphine is the standard strong analgesic used clinically but it acts on only one of the three opioid receptors. This receptor (the μ-receptor), also mediates the side effects of the drug, which can limit the dose used and so the degree of pain relief. There is hope that new drugs acting on the other receptors, the δ (delta) and κ (kappa), would provide pain relief without the same degree of side effects. (A fourth re-ceptor—the σ or sigma receptor—has also been described but is not considered to be a true opioid receptor.)

A summary chart (Fig. 18) on opioids, their receptors and their antagonists is given at the end of this chapter [see also Answer 28 in Part 2].

Drugs used clinically include: morphine, naloxone, pethidine, methadone, codeine, diamorphine (heroin), **fentanyl, bupre-norphine** and **pentazocine.**

QUESTIONS

1. What mediators act on peripheral nociceptive endings following tissue damage?

2. What transmitters are released at the central terminals of C-fibres?

3. Would local anaesthetics influence spinal transmitter release?

4. What are hyperalgesia and allodynia?

5. What spinal cord transmitters are thought to be involved in hyperalgesia and allodynia?

6. Has the sympathetic nervous system a role in pain?

7. Name the three main opioid receptors.

8. Name the three main endogenous opioids, indicating which receptor they act on.

9. For each opioid receptor, give an example of a clinically used drug acting mainly on that receptor.

10. Which drug is an antagonist at all opioid receptors?

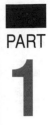

11. Name a drug which has partial agonist properties on an opioid receptor.

12. What are the differences between the terms 'opioid' and 'opiate'?

13. Name two agonists related in structure to **morphine**. Which one is found in opium?

14. **a.** What is the evidence for the interaction between **prostaglandins** and **bradykinin** on nociceptive afferent fibres?

    b. What might the clinical significance of this be?

15. Give an example of one of each of the four groups of synthetic derivatives with structures unrelated to **morphine**.

16. What happens to a neuron terminal when the opioid receptors are activated?

17. Give two main sites at which **morphine** acts to cause analgesia.

18. What are the main unwanted effects of **morphine** which occur at therapeutic doses?

19. **Morphine** can induce release of a mediator which produces itching, bronchoconstriction and hypotension. What is it and how does morphine release it?

20. What is the action of **morphine** on the respiratory centre? What is the basis for this action?

21. What pharmacological effects are associated with stimulation of the κ-opioid receptors as compared with μ- and δ-receptors?

22. Is **morphine** ever used therapeutically in the absence of pain?

23. **a.** What are the two main aspects of opiate dependence? What receptor is involved?

    b. Which **opiates** are considered to be less likely to cause dependence?

24. Why is **morphine** less active by the oral route?

25. What compound is produced when **codeine** or **heroin** is metabolised?

26. **a.** List the main pharmacological actions of **morphine**, specifying which are useful clinically.

    b. What is the basis for its action on GIT motility?

27. What is the advantage of intrathecal application of **morphine**?

28. In terms of the effect on the neonate, which drug, **morphine** or **pethidine**, might be preferred for analgesia during labour, and why?

29. Indicate whether the following statements are true or false. If you think a statement is false, explain why.

    a. A. Codeine has no addiction liability.

    B. Codeine is as potent an analgesic as morphine.

    C. In equiactive doses **codeine** produces less respiratory depression than **morphine**.

    D. Codeine is an effective analgesic for mild pain but its liability to cause constipation limits its long-term use.

    E. Dextropropoxyphene is an effective analgesic and has no dependence liability.

    F. Pethidine has antimuscarinic as well as opioid actions.

    G. Methadone is used in patient-controlled infusion systems because it has a short duration of action.

    H. Methadone is used with a neuroleptic to produce 'neuroleptanalgesia', a state in which some surgical operations can be performed without full anaesthesia.

    I. Etorphine is useful in the hippopotamus.

    J. Methadone is taken up and then slowly released from tissue stores.

K. Methadone is used to wean people off heroin.

L. Pentazocine is a μ-receptor agonist.

M. Pentazocine can cause dysphoria, nightmares and hallucinations.

N. Codeine can antagonise some actions of morphine and so cannot be given to people already on morphine.

O. Nalorphine is a mixed antagonist–agonist and can therefore both produce dependence and precipitate withdrawal, depending on the dose.

P. Naloxone is a pure competitive antagonist at all opioid receptors.

Q. Naloxone has a long half-life.

b. Morphine:

A. causes respiratory depression at therapeutic doses.

B. reduces the sensitivity of brain stem respiratory control areas to P_{CO_2}.

C. has, as its first effect on respiration, inhibition of the response of the chemoreceptors to hypoxia.

D. inhibits the cough reflex.

E. decreases GIT motility by decreasing smooth muscle tone in the intestine.

F. constricts the pupil by action on μ- and κ-receptors in the constrictor pupillae.

ANSWERS

1. **Bradykinin**, **prostanoids**, **5-HT**, **H⁺ ions** and **acetylcholine. Lactic acid**, **ATP** and **K⁺** may be involved in ischaemic pain [see 📖 pp. 614–615].

2. **Glutamate** and many peptides including **tachykinins** (of which **substance P** is a

member), **somatostatin**, **CGRP**, etc. Cooperation between these transmitters can lead to alterations in pain transmission [see 📖 pp. 615–616, 199–200].

3. Yes, but indirectly as a result of their block of conduction in a peripheral nerve [see 📖 Ch. 34].

4. Hyperalgesia is an enhanced response to a low level of noxious stimulation and allodynia is where touch is perceived as pain [see 📖 pp. 611].

5. The release of substance P and other peptides is believed to allow the NMDA receptor to be activated, which enhances and prolongs pain transmission. In addition, nitric oxide is produced from spinal neurons [see 📖 pp. 611].

6. Yes, but only in some types of neuropathic (nerve damage) pain where alpha-receptor-mediated excitation of nociceptive systems can occur [see 📖 p. 614].

7. μ, δ and κ. Although μ- and δ-receptors produce similar end effects they are clearly independent; delta opioids are as potent as morphine in producing analgesia [see 📖 p. 622 box].

8. β-endorphin (μ-receptor), enkephalins (δ-receptor) and dynorphin (κ-receptor) [see 📖 Table 31.3, p. 199].

9. μ-receptor: **morphine** (also **fentanyl**). δ-receptor: none as yet. κ-receptor: **pentazocine** (also cyclazocine) [see 📖 Table 31.3].

10. **Naloxone** (also **naltrexone**) [see 📖 Table 31.3].

11. **Nalorphine** and **pentazocine** are partial agonists on the κ-receptor; **buprenorphine** (also meptazinol) on the μ-receptor [see 📖 Table 31.3].

12. The differences are minimal: 'opioid' refers to substances with morphine-like

activity whether synthetic or endogenous peptides; whereas 'opiate' means drugs with structures similar to morphine [see ▱ p. 617].

13. Important examples are **heroin** and **codeine**, the latter being found in opium. There are others [see ▱ Table 31.1].

14. a. Prostaglandins (PGs) sensitise the nociceptive neuron by lowering its threshold of activation [see ▱ Fig. 31.5].

b. Such sensitisation accounts for a major part of the pain felt after surgery or trauma (**NSAIDs**, by inhibiting PG synthesis, may reduce such pain). But note that other agents (**leukotrienes**, **purines**) also sensitise the nociceptors.

15. Important examples are: **pethidine**, **fentanyl** (phenylpiperidines); **methadone**, **dextropropoxyphene** (methadone series); **pentazocine** (benzomorphan); **etorphine**, **buprenorphine** (thebaines) [see ▱ p. 619].

16. The terminal would be hyperpolarised since opiate receptors when activated open K$^+$ channels (μ and δ) or close calcium channels (κ). Thus neuronal activity will be decreased [see ▱ p. 622 box]. The shortening of the action potential due to the open K$^+$ or closed Ca^{2+} channels will reduce Ca^{2+} fluxes into the terminal. Less Ca^{2+} will mean less transmitter release from the terminals [see ▱ p. 621].

17. At supraspinal sites (involving the periaqueductal grey matter and raphe magnus) and in the spinal cord [see Fig. 18 and ▱ Fig. 31.4].

18. See Figure 18.

19. Morphine releases **histamine** from mast cells. It does this by virtue of the fact that it is a base, not by an action on opioid receptors.

20. Therapeutic doses of morphine depress the respiratory centre by an action on μ-

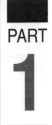

receptors. The response to P_{CO_2} is affected at lower concentrations than the hypoxic drive [see ▱ p. 623].

21. See Figure 18.

22. Yes. Firstly, it reduces anxiety and so when given preoperatively, prior to the production of pain, this effect will not only be helpful to the patient but the pre-emptive analgesic effect may also be useful. In addition, it is an excellent sedative and may be used to reduce anxiety in serious and frightening conditions not necessarily associated with pain, e.g. haematemesis (the vomiting of blood).*

23. a. Dependence can be psychological or physical; both can be produced with opiates, by action on μ-receptors [see ▱ p. 627 box].

b. Codeine, pentazocine, buprenorphine, nalbuphine [see p. 627 box].

24. Partly because it is a base, so it is ionised in the gut and trapped [see Fig. 4 in Ch. 4]. It is also subject to first-pass metabolism [see ▱ Table 4.3].

25. They are partly metabolised to **morphine**.

26. a. (i) Pain relief; (ii) sedation; (iii) euphoria; (iv) respiratory depression; (v) cough suppression; (vi) nausea and vomiting; (vii) reduced gastrointestinal motility; (viii) histamine release, which may cause bronchoconstriction and hypotension; (ix) pupillary constriction; (i), (v), and (vii) are clinically useful, also (ii), in some circumstances [see Answer 22 above and ▱ p. 624 box].

b. Morphine increases the tone and reduces the motility of the GIT. This is due partly to an inhibitory effect on the

---

* An excellent coverage of the clinical use of narcotic analgesics is given in Laurence D R, Bennett P N 1992 *Clinical Pharmacology*, 7th edn. Churchill Livingstone, Edinburgh.

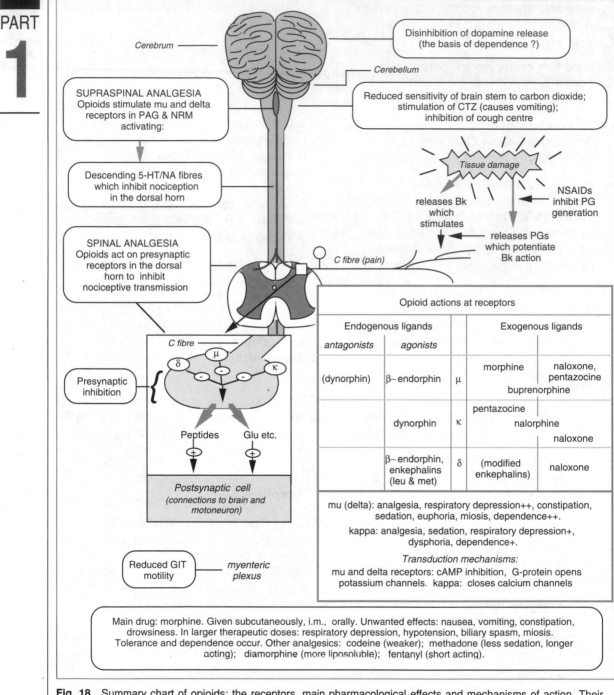

Fig. 18 Summary chart of opioids; the receptors, main pharmacological effects and mechanisms of action. Their interaction with NSAIDs is also shown. PAG = periaqueductal grey matter; NRM = nucleus raphe magnus; CTZ = chemoreceptor trigger zone; Bk = bradykinin; PG = prostaglandin.

myenteric plexus and partly to a central action. All three opioid receptors are involved [see 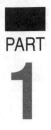 p. 624].

27. Spinal application is used to produce analgesia whilst avoiding the respiratory depression, dependence, etc, produced by action on brain sites, and the constipation produced by action in the GIT. This can be very useful during labour, and for the relief of postoperative pain and the pain of cancer.

28. **Pethidine** is generally preferred. If any pethidine given to the mother crosses to the neonate, it will be inactivated, whereas **morphine** will not. This is because morphine metabolism (but not pethidine metabolism) involves conjugation reactions which are deficient in the neonate [see 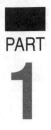 p. 629]. (But if spinal epidural injections of opiates are given, there can be good analgesia with little possibility of the drug crossing to the neonate.)

29. a. **A.** True in general; codeine rarely causes addiction.

   B. False; dose for dose it is only about 20% as potent and has a low ceiling of activity [see 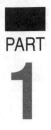 p. 629].

   C. False; at equiactive analgesic doses, **codeine** produces the same degree of respiratory depression as **morphine**, but codeine has a low ceiling of response so respiratory depression is not usually a problem at the doses used [see 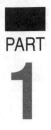 p. 629].

   D. True [see 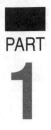 p. 629].

   E. False; it is now known to be less potent than **codeine** and it is not free of dependence liability [see 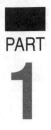 p. 629].

   F. True; it causes dry mouth and visual blurring [see 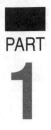 p. 629].

   G. False; **methadone** is long-acting. **Fentanyl** or **sufentanil**, both short-lasting, are used in patient-controlled

infusion analgesia [see 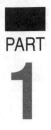 pp. 629, 630].

   H. False; **fentanyl** is short-acting (and potent) and so is used for neuroleptanalgesia; the effects wear off rapidly postoperatively [see 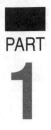 p. 630].

   I. True; it is used to tranquillise large wild beasts because it is so potent that a very large dose can be incorporated into a dart or pellet.

   J. True; this may be why it has a long duration of action [see 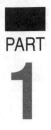 p. 630].

   K. True; the abstinence syndrome is less acute than with **morphine** [see 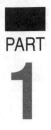 p. 630].

   L. False; it is an agonist at the κ-receptor but an antagonist at the μ-receptor [see 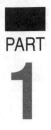 Table 31.3].

   M. True; it is not necessarily always that user-friendly.

   N. False; this is true for **pentazocine**, which is an antagonist, and **buprenorphine** which is a partial agonist on the μ-receptor [see 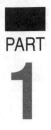 Table 31.3].

   O. True; at higher doses it has agonist properties [see 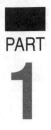 p. 630].

   P. True [see 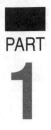 p. 631].

   Q. False; it is rapidly metabolised and is shorter-acting than most morphine-like drugs; infusions or repeated injections are often needed when it is used to overcome morphine overdose [see 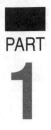 p. 631].

b. **Morphine**

   A. True [see 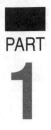 p. 623].

   B. True [see 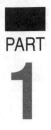 p. 623].

   C. False; the response to hypoxia is lost late. A patient with **morphine** overdose may be breathing only

PART

1

because of the hypoxic drive; if O$_2$ is given, without artificial ventilation, he/she may stop breathing altogether.

D. True [see 📖 p. 623].

E. False [see Answer 26b above].

F. False; pupillary constriction is due to action on μ- and κ-receptors in the oculomotor nucleus [see 📖 p. 624].

32

Central nervous system stimulants and psychotomimetic drugs

BACKGROUND INFORMATION

CNS stimulants fall into three groups: convulsants and respiratory stimulants, psychomotor stimulants and psychotomimetic drugs. The first group has little clinical use, except in the case of doxapram which is used to treat acute respiratory failure. The second category includes cocaine, amphetamine and caffeine. These are of considerable social importance since they are used for non-medical/recreational purposes by many individuals. They can produce euphoria, reduce fatigue and cause motor stimulation. Psychotomimetic drugs influence thought, perception and mood and include agents such as lysergic acid diethylamide, phencyclidine and cannabis.

Important drugs: doxapram, amphetamine, cocaine, theophylline, lysergic acid diethylamide, phencyclidine.

QUESTIONS

Convulsants and respiratory stimulants

1. What does the term 'analeptic' mean?

2. What are **amiphenazole** and **doxapram** used for?

3. On what receptor does **strychnine** act? Does it function as an agonist or an antagonist?

4. How do **a. bicuculline** and **b. picrotoxin** act?

Psychomotor stimulants

5. List the four main effects of the **amphetamines**.

6. **a.** In an experimental situation, what procedures would prevent **amphetamine** from producing stereotyped behaviour?

b. What does this indicate regarding the transmitter system acted on by **amphetamine**?

7. What does **amphetamine** psychosis resemble?

8. Name a clinical indication for the use of **amphetamine**.

9. What is the basis of the pharmacological action of **cocaine** in the CNS?

10. Is there a marked difference between the psychological effects of **cocaine** and **amphetamine** on an individual?

11. What is crack?

12. Do **cocaine** and **amphetamine** cause physical dependence?

Methylxanthines
13. Name two main agents in this class which have stimulant effects on the CNS.

14. What is the mechanism of action of the **methylxanthines**?

15. List the four main actions of the **methylxanthine** drugs.

16. What is the main clinical use of **theophylline**?

Psychotomimetic drugs
17. **a.** What does LSD stand for?

b. What are the effects of LSD?

c. Does physical dependence occur with LSD?

d. What is thought to be the mechanism of action of LSD?

e. What happens in a bad trip?

18. How does **phencyclidine** act?

19. Indicate whether the following statements are true or false. If you think a statement is false, explain why.

A. Cocaine increases NA release by blocking uptake 2.

B. Theophylline causes stimulation of cardiac muscle by inhibiting the phosphodiesterase which metabolises intracellular cAMP.

C. The improved mental performance produced by coffee is related to the antagonism by **caffeine** of the action of adenosine on A_1- and A_2-receptors in the CNS.

D. Some of the CNS effects of **amphetamines** are due to release of **dopamine**.

E. Some of the effects of **LSD** are due to inhibition of **5-HT** release.

F. Phencyclidine, which causes hallucinations, delusions and sensory changes, is structurally related to the clinically useful anaesthetic, **ketamine**.

ANSWERS

1. Analeptic is an old term for drugs used to treat coma or severe respiratory depression. There is little evidence for any maintained benefit [see 🔖 p. 634].

2. As respiratory stimulants; they carry less risk of producing convulsions than other compounds [see 🔖 p. 636 box].

3. It is an antagonist on the glycine receptor, acting mainly in the spinal cord and, since glycine is an inhibitory transmitter in the spinal cord, **strychnine** will cause increased reflex excitability [see 🔖 pp. 634–635, 514 box].

4. **Bicuculline** acts as a competitive antagonist at the $GABA_A$ receptor, and **picrotoxin** probably blocks the associated chloride channel [see Fig. 34 and 🔖 Table 32.1].

5. Locomotor stimulation, euphoria, stereotyped (i.e. repeated non-purposeful) behaviour and anorexia [see 🔖 p. 640 box].

6. **a.** Depletion of **noradrenaline** and **dopamine** from the brain, block of their

synthesis, destruction of the dopamine neurons in nucleus accumbens and the use of dopamine antagonists [see 🖋 p. 637].

b. Dopamine is thus likely to underlie many of the behavioural effects of amphetamine, with a contribution from noradrenaline [see 🖋 pp. 636–637].

7. Schizophrenia; **dopamine antagonists** can improve both [see 🖋 p. 638].

8. The treatment of hyperkinetic children (controversial, but used in some countries) and the therapy of narcolepsy. (Falling asleep whilst revising is not necessarily a symptom of narcolepsy.) You may have listed obesity; in fact, although **amphetamine** itself is an appetite suppressant, it is best avoided for obesity treatment. However, related compounds (**fenfluramine** or **dexfenfluramine**) may sometimes be used short term, with care, in therapy of extreme obesity. They seem to act by releasing 5-HT rather than NA [see 🖋 Table 32.2, p. 638, Fig. 32.2].

9. **Cocaine** blocks uptake 1, the process by which released noradrenaline is taken back into the nerve terminal; its effects will therefore be those associated with increased action of noradrenaline [see 🖋 p. 640 box].

10. No; subjects can rarely distinguish between the psychological effects of the two drugs [see 🖋 p. 639 box].

11. Crack is a preparation of the free base of cocaine.

12. No, but very strong psychological dependence occurs with both [see 🖋 p. 640 box].

13. **Caffeine** and **theophylline** [see 🖋 Table 32.1].

14. It is thought that they act by inhibiting the cAMP phosphodiesterase and so increase cAMP. In addition they may act

as adenosine antagonists [see 🖋 pp. 641 box, 360 box].

15. Relaxation of smooth muscle [see Fig. 22], stimulation of cardiac muscle, diuresis, CNS stimulation [see 🖋 Fig. 14.1, p. 641 box].

16. As a bronchodilator [see 🖋 pp. 360 box, 641 box].

17. **a.** Lysergic acid diethylamide.

b. Alterations of perception, hallucinations, confusion of sensory modalities [see 🖋 p. 642].

c. No, but psychological dependence does [see 🖋 p. 642].

d. There is evidence that in the CNS, LSD acts as an agonist at one of the 5-HT receptors, the 5-HT$_1$ autoreceptor. This decreases the release of 5-HT, which normally exerts an inhibiting influence on cortical neurons with resultant filtering of incoming sensory information; the consequent loss of control may produce the hallucinations [see 🖋 p. 643].

LSD also has a high affinity for dopamine D$_2$-receptors: this might be involved in its psychotropic actions.

e. LSD-induced paranoia and severe threatening hallucinations which can lead to suicide attempts [see 🖋 pp. 642, 643 box].

18. It interacts with the opioid sigma receptor and also blocks the NMDA receptor channel which is activated by glutamate [see 🖋 pp. 509, 643 box].

19. **A.** False; **cocaine** doesn't increase the release of NA. It increases the local 'pool' of released NA by blocking uptake 1, the mechanism for re-uptake into the noradrenergic neuron of released NA [see 🖋 p. 640 box].

B. True [see 🖋 p. 641].

C. True. Note that the xanthine drug, **enprophylline**, which does not have an adenosine antagonism, does not have any CNS actions [see 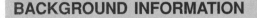 pp. 641, 360 box].

D. True [see ✍ p. 640 box].

E. True [see Answer 17d].

F. True; and **ketamine** can cause hallucinations during recovery from anaesthesia in some subjects [see ✍ pp. 546 box, 643].

33

Drug dependence and drug abuse

BACKGROUND INFORMATION

A number of drugs have no clinical uses but are consumed for social and recreational reasons. If one also considers the stimulant drugs (amphetamine and cocaine, Ch. 30) the opiates (Ch. 29) barbiturates and benzodiazepines (Ch. 25) and the LSD-like drugs (Ch. 30), a disparate group of pharmacologically active drugs emerges. Pharmacology cannot explain why one member of this group will be chosen for use as opposed to another; the social factors are of prime importance.

Drug dependence involves an obsessive craving for a drug after taking it repeatedly. It comprises:

- physical dependence (i.e. distinct symptoms are seen on withdrawal)
- tolerance (decreasing pharmacological effect with repeated administration)
- psychological dependence.

True physical dependence occurs mainly with the opiates and ethanol. Opiates are dealt with in Chapter 31.

Nicotine from tobacco has CNS and peripheral effects by action on nicotinic receptors and causes a mixture of stimulant and inhibitory responses. Tolerance and psychological and physical dependence result and the heavy prices to pay in terms of health are coronary disease, deleterious effects on foetal growth, and cancer of the respiratory tract. Nicotine and the CO generated during smoking are responsible for the first two conditions, tobacco-derived tars for the last.

Ethanol is a general depressant although lower doses cause the sought-after disinhibitory CNS effects. Tolerance and both physical and psychological dependence can occur, as can brain-cell death, liver cirrhosis and foetal abnor-

PART 1

malities. However, there is evidence that ischaemic heart disease is reduced in nationalities with moderate social drinking habits.

Cannabis was, until recently, little understood, since the depressant, euphoric and relaxant effects could not be attributed to any particular site of action. The recent isolation and cloning of a receptor should aid study of this agent. Little dependence is produced.

Important drugs: nicotine, ethanol, disulfiram, tetrahydrocannabinol.

QUESTIONS

1. Name the main categories of drugs with **a.** depressant, **b.** stimulant effects on the CNS which are subject to abuse.

2. **a.** Which of the above groups (depressant and stimulant drugs) are liable to cause psychological dependence?

   b. Which cause physical dependence?

3. What is the pharmacologically active substance in tobacco?

4. **a.** What are the effects of nicotine on the CNS?

   b. What are the effects of nicotine on the PNS?

   c. How rapid is the absorption of nicotine? What is its $t_{1/2}$?

   d. What types of dependence occur with nicotine?

   e. What are the health problems associated with smoking and what in tobacco causes them?

5. **a.** What is a unit of alcohol?

   b. What is the alcohol content of beer and of whisky?

   c. What does alcohol do to the CNS?

   d. What mechanisms are involved in the action of alcohol on the CNS?

   e. Does alcohol cause brain damage?

6. Indicate whether the following statements about ethanol are true or false. If you think a statement is false, explain why.

   A. It causes vasoconstriction.

   B. It can cause gastritis.

   C. It causes diuresis.

   D. It can cause liver damage.

   E. It is a useful food source.

   F. It can protect against ischaemic heart disease.

   G. It can damage foetuses.

   H. The more of it you drink, the more rapidly it is metabolised.

   I. It is metabolised to acetaldehyde.

   J. Tolerance, and both psychological and physical dependence occur with it.

7. **a.** What is the active agent in cannabis?

   b. What are the central effects of the drug?

   c. What are the peripheral effects?

   d. Is dependence marked?

ANSWERS

1. **a.** Opiates, alcohol, barbiturates and solvents.

   b. Cocaine, amphetamine, nicotine and caffeine.

2. **a.** Both, hence the craving or desire to take them.

   b. Only the depressants cause physical dependence.

3. Nicotine, acting on CNS nicotinic receptors [see 🖉 p. 651 box].

4. **a.** Generally, an alerting effect in relaxed subjects and a depressant effect when tense. EEG recordings clearly show this biphasic effect, which may depend on dose. Learning and vigilance often improve [see 🖉 p. 651 box].

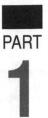

b. Stimulation of autonomic ganglia, and secretion of adrenaline and ADH. Tolerance occurs to these effects [see 🖎 p. 651 box].

c. It is very rapidly absorbed from the lungs (cigarettes) and mouth and nasopharynx (pipes). The $t_{1/2}$ is about 10 minutes initially but due to redistribution a slow decline then follows.

d. Both strong psychological and some physical dependence result; withdrawal symptoms include sleep disturbances and irritability.

e. Lung cancer (tars); other cancers (tars); ischaemic heart disease (nicotine and CO); bronchitis (tars); foetal weight reduction and development (nicotine and CO) [see 🖎 p. 653 box].

5. **a.** About 8g of ethanol, equivalent to a glass of wine, a measure of spirits or half a pint of beer.

b. About 2–5% for beers and lagers, up to 55% for strong spirits.

c. Depresses all systems, although at low doses it may inhibit inhibitory systems and this disinhibition may be the basis for the increased social confidence seen at low levels of drinking. Impairment increases with increasing dosage, finally leading to coma [see 🖎 pp. 654–655].

d. Many theories are proposed including a general membrane action, reduced transmitter release, inhibition of Ca^{2+} entry, antagonism of excitatory amino acid effects and enhancement of GABA actions. Since no receptor is involved, the overall effects probably include many if not all of these [see 🖎 pp. 654–655].

e. Yes, heavy drinkers may have cerebellar and hippocampal damage [see 🖎 p. 655].

6. **A.** False; it causes vasodilatation which causes a feeling of warmth, but heat is lost. St Bernard dogs may have a lot to answer for.

B. True; heavy drinkers usually have damaged gastric mucosa.

C. True; it inhibits ADH secretion which, together with the volume of liquid imbibed, combines to cause queuing for the bathroom at parties.

D. True; due to impaired oxidation of fat (and increased release of fatty acids from adipose tissue), fat builds up in the liver which progresses eventually to cirrhosis.

E. False; it provides calories but no vitamins, cofactors, amino acids or fats.

F. This is true; but only for moderate consumption, which is said to result in increased HDL levels [see 🖎 Ch. 15].

G. True; it can produce the foetal alcohol syndrome (facial malformation, growth and development problems, etc) [see 🖎 p. 657].

H. False; metabolism follows zero-order kinetics, so as the concentration increases so does the duration of effect [see 🖎 Figs 33.5, 4.24].

I. True; disulfiram blocks further metabolism and so causes adverse effects due to build up of the acetaldehyde [see 🖎 Fig. 33.4].

J. True.

7. **a.** Cannabinols, of which there are several variants with Δ^1- THC being the most important. We may have to add anandamide, which could be the endogenous cannabis transmitter.

b. It causes relaxation and a sense of well-being, together with some degree of increased sensory activity. A mild general impairment of performance has been noted [see 🖎 p. 663 box].

c. Tachycardia, vasodilatation, reduced ocular pressure, bronchodilatation and an inhibition of nausea.

d. No.

34

Local anaesthetics and other drugs that affect excitable membranes

BACKGROUND INFORMATION

Electrical excitability of the membranes of nerve and muscle allows the generation of action potentials. Voltage-dependent Na^+ channels and to a lesser extent K^+ channels control this excitability. Local anaesthetics and also phenytoin, some neurotoxins such as tetrodotoxin, and K^+ channel agents all have influences on these events. The sensory receptors on peripheral sensory nerve terminals and on postsynaptic membranes initiate depolarisation and generate action potentials. The action potential consists of a self-propagating depolarisation which passes rapidly along the nerve fibre. The basis of this is the opening of voltage-operated Na^+ channels, the inward Na^+ current causing further membrane depolarisation. The depolarisation also initiates the opening of K^+ channels. The outward K^+ current, along with the closure of the Na^+ channels (termed inactivation), results in repolarisation.

Local anaesthetics act by blocking the voltage-dependent Na^+ channels. The side effects of local anaesthetics are mainly due to their escape into the circulation. Local anaesthetics can be applied by a variety of routes including surface application to mucous membranes, infiltration, regional block via intravenous administration in the presence of a cuff and direct spinal application. (K^+ channel blockers are being explored for clinical use).

Important drugs: procaine, lignocaine, bupivacaine and **prilocaine**.

A summary chart of local anaesthetics (Fig. 19) is given on page 116.

QUESTIONS

1. **a.** What is the difference in the time course of the Na^+ and K^+ conductances during the action potential?

    b. What is the direction of ion flow in the two cases?

    c. What membrane changes are associated with the rising phase of the action potential?

    d. What is the refractory period?

    e. What membrane changes are associated with the decay of the action potential (i.e. the recovery of the membrane potential)?

2. What is the basic structure of voltage-gated ion channels?

3. **a.** How can drugs decrease membrane excitability in neurons?

    b. Is it possible to increase neuronal membrane excitability? If so, how?

4. What is the basic structure of a local anaesthetic?

5. From which side of the neuronal membrane do most local anaesthetics act?

6. Give examples of drugs that act on each (not both) of the following:

    a. the heart

    b. the CNS

    by a mechanism of action similar to that of the local anaesthetics.

7. Describe the mechanism by which local anaesthetics block action potential generation.

8. What is use-dependence?

9. What is the order of block produced by local anaesthetics on peripheral nerve fibre types?

10. What unwanted effects could occur if local anaesthetics gain access to the CNS?

11. How does **cocaine** differ from the other local anaesthetics in terms of its actions on the CNS?

12. What unwanted cardiovascular effects occur if local anaesthetics escape into the circulation?

13. How are local anaesthetics metabolised?

14. Name two local anaesthetics that are best suited for surface administration to mucous membranes.

15. **a.** What is infiltration anaesthesia?

    b. Why are **adrenaline** or **felypressin** added to local anaesthetics for infiltration anaesthesia?

16. What is nerve block anaesthesia?

17. What is spinal anaesthesia and what are the main advantages and disadvantages of the technique?

18. Why should you be wary of inadequately prepared puffer fish and chips on the canteen menu?

19. Name three types of K⁺ channels.

20. Would **lignocaine** have greater or lesser action in infected tissue? Give reasons for your answer.

ANSWERS

1. **a.** The rise in K⁺ conductance occurs later than the rise in Na⁺ conductance.

    b. Na⁺ ions flow inwards, K⁺ ions move outwards.

    c. The increase in Na⁺ permeability, resulting in inward Na⁺ current.

    d. The refractory period, during which the cell is inexcitable, is the time during which many Na⁺ channels are inactivated, and the K⁺ conductance is raised.

    e. The opening of voltage-operated K⁺ channels and the inactivation of Na⁺ channels [see 🖊 p. 669 box].

2. Each channel consists of four protein domains, each domain consisting of six membrane-spanning α-helices. The four domains are arranged round a central pore, which forms the ion channel.

3. **a.** By blocking Na⁺ channels. The **local anaesthetics** have this action as do

certain neurotoxins used as experimental tools (**tetrodotoxin**, **saxotoxin**) [see 🖊 p. 669 box].

    b. Yes, by blocking K⁺ channels (e.g. **tetraethylammonium**) or by inhibiting the inactivation of Na⁺ channels (e.g. **veratridine**) [see 🖊 p. 669 box, Figs 34.3, 34.5].

4. An aromatic moiety which is joined by an ester or amide bond to a basic side chain [see Fig. 19 and 🖊 Fig. 34.5].

5. The inner side [see Fig. 19 and 🖊 p. 671 box].

6. **a.** Class I antidysrhythmic drugs, e.g. **quinidine**, **flecainide**.

    b. The antiepileptic drug, **phenytoin** [see 🖊 Table 13.1, p. 665].

7. They block Na⁺ channels directly. With most local anaesthetics, the unionised species penetrates the axonal membrane. Within the axoplasm the molecule becomes charged and the ionised species blocks the sodium channels. With some local anaesthetics, the unionised species can enter the channel directly from the membrane [see Fig. 19 and 🖊 Fig. 34.6].

8. In simple terms, the greater the frequency of action potentials, the greater the channel block, since the channels are open more often and inactivate more often, and **local anaesthetics** gain access to the channels more readily when they are open and have higher affinity for inactivated than resting channels [see 🖊 p. 671 box, Fig. 34.6].

9. Nociceptive and sympathetic fibres first, followed by temperature, then touch and pressure, then proprioception and motor nerves—in that order [see Fig. 19 and 🖊 pp. 671–672].

10. Generally activation, causing restlessness, tremor, leading to confusion and convulsions. Procaine is the most likely to cause these problems [see 🖊 p. 672].

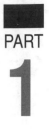

PART

1

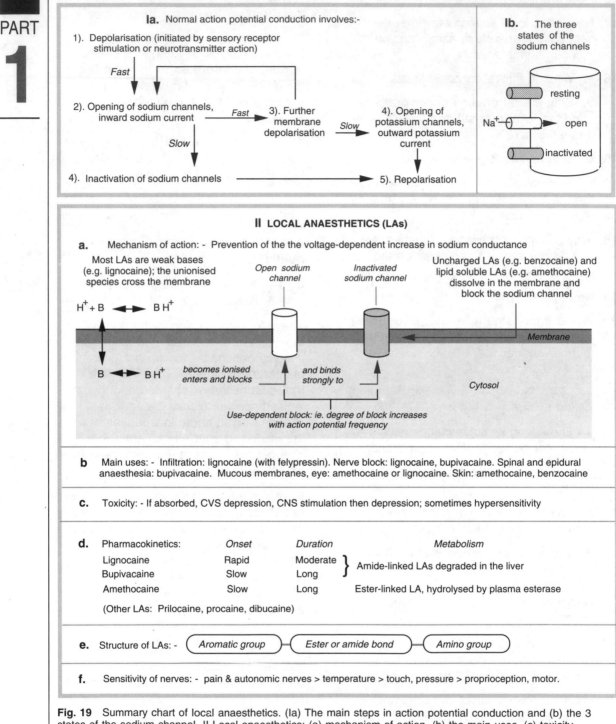

Ia. Normal action potential conduction involves:-

1). Depolarisation (initiated by sensory receptor stimulation or neurotransmitter action)

Fast

2). Opening of sodium channels, inward sodium current → *Fast* → 3). Further membrane depolarisation → *Slow* → 4). Opening of potassium channels, outward potassium current

Slow

4). Inactivation of sodium channels ⟶ 5). Repolarisation

Ib. The three states of the sodium channels

Na^+ — resting / open / inactivated

II LOCAL ANAESTHETICS (LAs)

a. Mechanism of action: - Prevention of the the voltage-dependent increase in sodium conductance

Most LAs are weak bases (e.g. lignocaine); the unionised species cross the membrane

Open sodium channel   *Inactivated sodium channel*

Uncharged LAs (e.g. benzocaine) and lipid soluble LAs (e.g. amethocaine) dissolve in the membrane and block the sodium channel

$H^+ + B \leftrightarrow BH^+$

Membrane

$B \leftrightarrow BH^+$

becomes ionised enters and blocks   *and binds strongly to*   *Cytosol*

Use-dependent block: ie. degree of block increases with action potential frequency

b. Main uses: - Infiltration: lignocaine (with felypressin). Nerve block: lignocaine, bupivacaine. Spinal and epidural anaesthesia: bupivacaine. Mucous membranes, eye: amethocaine or lignocaine. Skin: amethocaine, benzocaine

c. Toxicity: - If absorbed, CVS depression, CNS stimulation then depression; sometimes hypersensitivity

d. Pharmacokinetics:

	Onset	Duration	Metabolism
Lignocaine	Rapid	Moderate	} Amide-linked LAs degraded in the liver
Bupivacaine	Slow	Long	
Amethocaine	Slow	Long	Ester-linked LA, hydrolysed by plasma esterase

(Other LAs: Prilocaine, procaine, dibucaine)

e. Structure of LAs: - (Aromatic group)—(Ester or amide bond)—(Amino group)

f. Sensitivity of nerves: - pain & autonomic nerves > temperature > touch, pressure > proprioception, motor.

Fig. 19 Summary chart of local anaesthetics. (Ia) The main steps in action potential conduction and (b) the 3 states of the sodium channel. II Local anaesthetics: (a) mechanism of action, (b) the main uses, (c) toxicity, (d) pharmacokinetic aspects, (e) an outline of the basic structure and (f) the differential sensitivity of different nerves.

11. In addition to its local anaesthetic activity, **cocaine** blocks monoamine uptake 1, so increasing synaptic monoamines and causing stimulation [see 📖 p. 672].

12. Myocardial depression and vasodilatation [see 📖 p. 673 box].

13. Plasma cholinesterase cleaves the ester-linked anaesthetics; the amide-linked compounds are metabolised in the liver, often to active metabolites [see 📖 pp. 672–673].

14. You could have named **lignocaine, tetracaine, dibucaine, cocaine** [see 📖 Table 34.2]. (Cocaine is rarely used now.)

15. **a.** Injection of local anaesthetic into tissues to anaesthetise sensory nerve terminals and fine nerve branches [see 📖 Table 34.2].

    b. To produce vasoconstriction which will limit vascular reabsorption of the drug, so increasing local concentration and reducing the amount required and the possibility of systemic toxicity [see 📖 Table 34.2].

16. Injection of the anaesthetic close to a nerve trunk. This involves considerably less anaesthetic than for infiltration anaesthesia [see 📖 Table 34.2].

17. Spinal anaesthesia is the application of local anaesthetic directly onto the spinal cord or onto the dura. This localisation allows low doses to be used, whereas the area anaesthetised can be quite extensive. Thus, e.g. the repair of hernias or pelvic surgery can be carried out under spinal anaesthesia in a conscious (but sedated) patient. Disadvantages are:

    (i) that there is block of the preganglionic sympathetic fibres, which are affected by lower concentrations of local anaesthetic than are sensory or somatic motor nerves

    (ii) that longitudinal spread may cause unwanted effects [see 📖 Table 34.2].

18. Because it may contain **tetrodotoxin**, a Na^+ channel blocker [see 📖 p. 673].

19. Voltage-activated, calcium-activated and ATP-sensitive [see 📖 p. 676].

20. **Lignocaine**, like most local anaesthetics, is a weak base with a pKa of 8–9. In an area of infection the pH of the extracellular fluid is usually lower than the normal pH of 7.4; consequently there might be less unionised drug and thus less penetration of the local anaesthetic into the nerve.

PART

1

117

35

Basic principles of chemotherapy

BACKGROUND INFORMATION

To be effective, chemotherapeutic agents should be maximally toxic for invading pathogenic organisms and innocuous for host cells. This can be accomplished if there are exploitable biochemical differences between the invading organism and the host.

Taking the bacterial cell as an example of an invading organism, one can delineate three general classes of biochemical reactions as potential targets for chemotherapy as follows:

Class I reactions in which glucose or other carbon sources are used both for energy generation and to make simple carbon compounds which are precursors for:

Class II reactions in which energy and class I compounds are used to make small molecules such as amino acids, nucleotides, etc, for:

Class III reactions in which these small molecules are built into macromolecules such as peptidoglycan, proteins, nucleic acids, polysaccharides.

Class I reactions provide no worthwhile targets for chemotherapy, class II reactions offer a few, class III reactions provide the majority.

QUESTIONS

1. What drugs interfere with folate synthesis in bacteria and how do they do this?

2. Name three drugs which interfere with folate utilisation specifically in:
   a. bacteria; **b.** malarial parasites;
   c. humans?

3. Name three chemotherapeutic agents which can interfere with peptidoglycan synthesis.

4. Name three chemotherapeutic agents which can interfere with bacterial protein synthesis.

5. Name three chemotherapeutic agents which can inhibit nucleic acid synthesis. What microorganisms, parasites, cell types, etc, are affected by the agents specified?

6. How is drug resistance spread among bacteria?

7. Give an example of a chemotherapeutic agent which acts by interfering with nucleotide synthesis in: **a.** a cancer cell; **b.** a fungal cell.

8. What are promiscuous plasmids?

9. List the main biochemical mechanisms of resistance to antibiotics.

10. So-called '**methicillin-resistant**' staphylococci manifest resistance to many other antibiotics. List three and specify the basis of the resistance.

11. Indicate which of the following statements are true and which false. If you think a statement is false, explain why.

   A. Sulphonamides are bacteriostatic.

   B. Penicillin is bactericidal.

   C. Streptomycin interferes with peptidoglycan synthesis.

   D. The chemotherapeutic action of **4-quinolone antibacterials** is due to inhibition of DNA gyrase.

   E. The antibacterial action of **polymixin** antibiotics is due to inhibition of protein synthesis.

   F. Rifampicin acts against the tubercle bacillus by inhibiting its protein synthesis.

   G. Adenosine arabinoside has antiviral activity by altering the base-pairing properties of the DNA.

   H. Plasmids are extra-chromosomal loops of DNA which can replicate entirely on their own.

   I. In the context of the transfer of resistance to antibiotics between

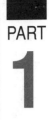

bacteria, transduction involves transfer of plasmid DNA from one bacterium to another by means of sex pili.

J. Sulphonamide-resistance is due to the production of β-lactamase with low affinity for sulphonamides.

ANSWERS

1. **Sulphonamides**: by competing with pABA for the enzyme involved in bacterial folate synthesis [see 📖 p. 683].

2. Three drugs which interfere with folic acid utilisation in **a.** bacteria, **b.** malarial parasites and **c.** humans are: (i) **trimethoprim**, (ii) **pyrimethamine** and (iii) **methotrexate** respectively [see 📖 pp. 683, 690 box].

3. The most important group are the lactam antibiotics (**penicillins, cephalosporins, monobactams, carbapenems**). Others are **vancomycin, cycloserine, bacitracin** [see 📖 Fig. 35.3].

4. **Tetracyclines**, the **aminoglycosides, chloramphenicol, erythromycin, fusidic acid, spectinomycin** (all used clinically) and **puromycin** (an investigatory tool) [see 📖 Fig. 35.4].

5. Antibacterials: **rifampicin, rifamycin**, the 4-quinolones (e.g. ciprofloxacin);

    Antivirals: **acyclovir, adenine arabinoside**;

    Antimalarials: **chloroquine**;

    Anticancer agents: **cytarabine**, nitrogen mustards (e.g. **cyclophosphamide**), **nitrosoureas, dactinomycin**;

    Antischistosome agents: **hycanthone**;

    Antiseptics: **proflavine, acriflavine**;

    [see 📖 pp. 688–689].

6. There are three mechanisms: the transfer of resistance genes through sex pili (i.e. conjugation); the transfer of resistance genes by a phage (i.e. transduction); the

taking up of naked DNA (i.e. transformation). The first is the most important, the last the least important [see 📖 pp. 693 box, 692].

7. **a. Fluorouracil, thioguanine, mercaptopurine**.

    b. Flucytosine.

    [See 📖 p. 684.]

8. Not what you think they are. The term refers to conjugative plasmids that code for sex pili, but does not apply to all of these—only to those that can cross the barriers between different species of bacteria [see 📖 p. 692].

9. (i) Production of enzymes that inactivate the drug, e.g. β-lactamases (inactivate **penicillin**), acetyltransferases (inactivate **chloramphenicol**), kinases, etc (inactivate **aminoglycosides**).

    (ii) Alteration of drug-binding site in microorganism for **penicillin, aminoglycosides, erythromycin**.

    (iii) Reduction of drug uptake by the bacterium, e.g. **tetracyclines**.

    (iv) Alteration in bacterial enzyme, e.g. dihydrofolate reductase becomes insensitive to **trimethoprim**.

    [See 📖 pp. 693–695.]

10. Methicillin-resistant staphylococci may also manifest resistance to **streptomycin, aminoglycosides, chloramphenicol**, the **macrolides, trimethoprim, sulphonamides, rifampicin, fusidic acid** [see 📖 p. 694].

11. **A.** True [see 📖 pp. 683–684].

    B. True; it results in lysis of susceptible bacteria.

    C. False; its primary action is interference with protein synthesis by causing abnormal codon:anticodon recognition [see 📖 Fig. 35.4].

    D. True [see 📖 p. 689].

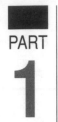

E. False; **polymixins** interact with phospholipids in the cell membrane and cause lysis [see 🕮 pp. 689–690].

F. False: **rifampicin** inhibits bacterial RNA polymerase [see 🕮 p. 689].

G. True [see 🕮 p. 688].

H. False; they can only replicate within bacteria, but do so independently of the bacterial DNA [see 🕮 p. 691].

I. False; transduction is the transfer of plasmid DNA by an 'infection' process by bacterial virus [see 🕮 p. 692].

J. False; **sulphonamide** resistance is due to production of a dihydropteroate synthetase with low affinity for sulphonamides [see 🕮 p. 694].

36
Cancer chemotherapy

BACKGROUND INFORMATION

The term 'cancer' refers to a malignant neoplasm (new growth). Cancer cells manifest, in greater or lesser degree:

- uncontrolled proliferation
- invasiveness
- the ability to metastasise.

Benign neoplasms manifest only uncontrolled proliferation.

The two main DNA changes underlying cancerous change in a cell are:

- inactivation of tumour-suppressor genes
- activation of proto-oncogenes (genes normally involved in cell growth and differentiation) to oncogenes.

Most anticancer agents are mainly, if not entirely, antiproliferative and will also affect rapidly dividing normal cells.

Drugs used clinically are:
Alkylating agents, e.g. **cyclophosphamide, carmustine**
Antimetabolites, e.g. **methotrexate, cytarabine**
Cytotoxic antibiotics, e.g. **doxorubicin, bleomycin**
Plant alkaloids, e.g. **vincristine, etoposide**
Hormones, e.g. **glucocorticoids, sex hormones**
Radioactive isotopes, e.g. ^{131}**I**
Miscellaneous agents, e.g. **crisantaspase, procarbazine.**

QUESTIONS

1. What is the mechanism of action of the **alkylating agents**?

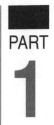

2. How is **cyclophosphamide** activated in the body to give rise to cytotoxic anticancer metabolite(s)?

3. The anticancer agent **a.** .... is taken up by cells by the transport system used by folate, and within the cell the agent is metabolised to **b.** ....

4. .... is an anticancer agent of low myelotoxicity which cross-links N7 to O6 of adjacent guanine molecules in the DNA in a manner analogous to the action of **cyclophosphamide**.

5. How does **methotrexate** exert its cytotoxic effect within a cancer cell?

6. What is the mechanism of action of **doxorubicin**?

7. The anticancer agent **a.** .... gives rise to a metabolite which can cause bladder damage that can be alleviated by infusing **b.** .... into the bladder by irrigation.

8. What are the mechanisms by which cancer cells can become resistant to: **a. methotrexate; b. alkylating agents; c. doxorubicin**?

9. What is the value of using combinations of anticancer drugs in cancer treatment?

10. Which anticancer drug(s) readily cross the blood–brain barrier and can therefore be used to treat tumours in the CNS?

11. What are the main general toxic actions of cytotoxic anticancer drugs?

12. What is the basis of multidrug resistance to anticancer drugs?

13. Indicate which of the following statements are true and which false. If you think a statement is false, explain why.

    A. Busulphan has a pronounced action against lymphocytes and can therefore be used as an immunosuppressant.

    B. Fluorouracil has a higher affinity than endogenous dihydrofolate for dihydrofolate reductase.

    C. Cytarabine is phosphorylated to the triphosphate which then inhibits DNA polymerase.

    D. Methotrexate reaches high concentrations in the CNS and can be used in the therapy of brain tumours.

    E. Vincristine's unwanted actions affect mainly neural tissue.

    F. Bleomycin, which has low myelotoxicity, can usefully be used with drugs which are myelosuppressive, in combination treatment regimes.

    G. Mercaptopurine has anticancer cytotoxic activity because it interferes with topoisomerase II.

    H. The most serious toxic effect of **crisantaspase** is pulmonary fibrosis.

14. Indicate which of the following anticancer agents, if any, do not cause severe myelotoxicity: **cisplatin, thioguanine, methotrexate, carboplatin, bleomycin**.

15. Indicate which of the following anticancer agents, if any, cause dose-limiting nephrotoxicity: **methotrexate, cisplatin, cytarabine, doxorubicin, etoposide**.

16. Which of the following anticancer agents, if any, can cause cumulative, dose-related cardiac damage: **cyclophosphamide, chlorambucil, doxorubicin, cytarabine, vincristine**.

ANSWERS

1. They form covalent bonds with DNA (mainly N7 of guanine); the inter- and intrastrand linking interfere with replication and transcription. Breakage of the chain and substitution of AT for GC can occur [see 📖 p. 706 box, Figs 36.3, 36.4].

2. It is activated to aldophosphamide, which is converted to phosphoramide mustard (the cytotoxic moiety) [see 📖 Fig. 36.6].

3. **a. Methotrexate; b.** methotrexate polyglutamate [see 📖 p. 708 box].

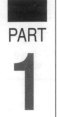

PART

1

4. **Cisplatin** [see 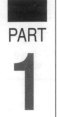 p. 706 box].

5. It inhibits dihydrofolate reductase and interferes with thymidylate synthesis [see p. 708 box, Figs 36.7, 36.8].

6. It intercalates in the DNA and interferes with the action of topoisomerase II [see p. 710 box].

7. a. **Cyclophosphamide**; b. **mesna** [see p. 706 box].

8. a. **Methotrexate**: decreased uptake, increased or modified dihydrofolate reductase, decreased polyglutamation of the drug.

   b. Alkylating agents: increased action of cancer cell DNA repair enzymes.

   c. Doxorubicin: modified cancer cell topoisomerase II.

   All may be affected by increased efflux due to multidrug resistance [see Answer 12 below].

9. Therapeutic but not toxic effects can be additive; the risk of resistance is lessened [see p. 713].

10. Nitrosoureas are the important ones, e.g. **carmustine**, **lomustine**, **semustine** [see p. 706 box]. **Fluorouracil**, **cytarabine**, **hydroxyurea** and **procarbazine** can also cross the blood–brain barrier.

11. Nausea and vomiting, myelotoxicity, decreased wound healing, depression of growth, sterility, teratogenicity, loss of hair [see p. 700 box].

12. Increased expression of a normal transport protein, P-glycoprotein, which causes increased *efflux* of anticancer drugs [see pp. 712–713].

13. **A.** False; this is true for **cyclophosphamide** [see p. 706 box].

   B. False; this is true for **methotrexate** [see p. 707].

   C. True [see p. 708 box].

   D. False; it has low lipid solubility and does not readily cross the blood–brain barrier [see p. 707].

E. True [see p. 710].

F. True [see p. 713].

G. False; this statement is true for **doxorubicin** and possibly for **etoposide**; **mercaptopurine** is converted into a 'fraudulent nucleotide' [see pp. 710 box, 708 box].

H. False; this statement is true for **bleomycin** (pulmonary fibrosis has also been reported to occur in patients treated with **bulsuphan**) [see pp. 710 box, 712].

14. **Cisplatin** and **bleomycin** do not cause severe myelotoxicity [see pp. 706 box, 710 box].

15. **Cisplatin** is concentrated in the kidney and can be seriously nephrotoxic. **Methotrexate**, in high dosage regimes, is also nephrotoxic [see pp. 706 box, 707].

16. **Doxorubicin** [see p. 709].

37

Antibacterial agents

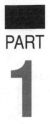

BACKGROUND INFORMATION

Most of the general background information is given in Chapter 35.

Drugs used clinically include:
Agents interfering with the synthesis action of folate: **sulphonamides, trimethoprim**
Beta-lactam antibiotics: **penicillins, cephalosporins, new β-lactamase-resistant β-lactam antibiotics**
Agents acting on bacterial protein synthesis: **tetracyclines, chloramphenicol, aminoglycosides, erythromycin**
Agents affecting topoisomerase II (DNA gyrase): 4-quinolones (e.g. **ciprofloxacin**)
Antituberculosis agents: **rifampicin, ethambutol, pyrazinamide, capreomycin, cycloserine**
Antileprosy agents: **dapsone, clofazimine**.

Factors to be considered in the choice of antibacterial agent are:

- the nature of the infecting organism and its sensitivity to antimicrobial drugs
- ability of the chosen agent to reach the target site
- possible evidence of previous hypersensitivity (allergy) to the chosen agent
- interactions of the agent with any other drugs the patient is taking
- possible increase in unwanted reactions to chosen agents due to host factors, e.g. age, renal impairment, liver disease, pregnancy, compromised immune system.

QUESTIONS

1. What is the mechanism of action of the **sulphonamides**?

2. The cell walls of Gram .... organisms consist of multiple layers (up to 40) of peptidoglycan.

3. It is necessary for patients on **sulphonamides** to take plenty of fluids because ....

4. Part of the chemical structure of the chemotherapy agent .... has some structural resemblance to the pteridine moiety of folate.

5. What are the main categories of **penicillin** antibiotics?

6. Outline the bacterial spectrum of **benzylpenicillin**.

7. Name: **a.** two broad-spectrum penicillins; **b.** two β-lactamase-resistant penicillins; **c.** one penicillin with spectrum extended to include pseudomonads.

8. What are the main steps in the antibacterial action of **penicillin** against susceptible Gram-positive organisms?

9. Define: **a** bacteriostatic; **b.** bactericidal.

10. Name two antibacterial agents whose action is bacteriostatic and two which are bactericidal.

11. What are the main mechanisms by which organisms become resistant to **benzylpenicillin**?

12. Since the introduction of **penicillin**, resistance of **a.** .... (give names of the types of bacteria) due to **b.** .... (give mechanism of resistance) has increased prodigiously, occurring particularly in hospitals. One technique of dealing with infections with these organisms is the concomitant use of **c.** .... (name drug), whose action is **d.** ....

13. Do the **penicillins** cross the blood–brain barrier?

14. How is **benzylpenicillin** given? What is its $t_{1/2}$?

15. What are the main categories of **cephalosporins**?

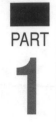

PART

1

16. Name a **cephalosporin** which is effective against pseudomonads.

17. .... is a non-penicillin, non-cephalosporin β-lactam antibiotic which has a broad antibacterial spectrum (including many aerobic and anaerobic Gram-positive and Gram-negative organisms) and high resistance to β-lactamases.

18. .... is a monocyclic β-lactam antibiotic, resistant to most β-lactamases, inactive against Gram-positive organisms, but active against Gram-negative rods.

19. Penicillin was originally termed 'the queen of drugs' because, due to its mode of action, it was considered to have no action at all on human cells and therefore to be totally non-toxic. Serious unwanted effects have since been recorded. What is the basis of these effects?

20. An important unwanted effect of the antibacterial agent .... is pancytopenia (a decrease in all blood cell elements), which can occur even with very low doses in some patients.

21. Outline the mechanism of antibacterial action of: **a.** the **tetracyclines**; **b. chloramphenicol**; **c.** the **aminoglycosides**; **d. erythromycin**.

22. .... must not be used in newborn babies, because inadequate activation and excretion may result in the 'grey baby' syndrome which has 40% mortality.

23. Antibacterial compounds of the .... group chelate metal ions; their absorption from the GIT is thus decreased in the presence of milk and antacids, and they may be deposited in growing bone.

24. Serious dose-related toxic effects involving the cochlea or vestibular organ of the ear and/or renal damage can occur with the antibacterial compounds ....

25. List: **a.** the first-line; **b.** the second-line drugs used to treat tuberculosis.

26. a. What is the mode of action of the **4-quinolone antimicrobial agents**?

b. Give two examples of this group of drugs.

27. What is the probable mechanism of action of **dapsone**?

28. What is **rifampicin** used for?

29. Outline the antibacterial spectrum of **ciprofloxacin**.

30. A patient with chronic congestive heart failure, who is being treated with **frusemide** plus **spironolactone** plus **captopril**, develops a severe urinary tract infection. The organisms are found to be sensitive to **trimethoprim**, **gentamycin**, **ciprofloxacin** and **cephradoxil**. Which antibacterial agent would you not use and why? (You can reach a sensible conclusion if you know the unwanted effects of the specified antibacterial agents.)

31. .... is an orally active drug effective against pseudomonads.

32. Indicate whether the following statements are true or false. If you think a statement is false, explain why.

A. Chloramphenicol is deposited in growing bones and teeth.

B. Tetracylines have a restricted antibacterial spectrum, confined mainly to Gram-negative bacteria.

C. Vancomycin is bactericidal, disrupting bacterial cell membranes by interaction with phospholipids.

D. Elimination of most **penicillins** is renal and occurs by glomerular filtration.

E. Plasma concentrations of the **aminoglycosides** should be carefully monitored because of the potential for dose-related nephrotoxicity and ototoxicity.

F. Erythromycin has the same antibacterial spectrum as penicillin and can be a useful alternative in patients allergic to penicillin.

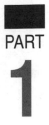

G. Cilastatin is a β-lactamase inhibitor used in combination with amoxycillin.

ANSWERS

1. They compete with pABA and thus interfere with bacterial folate synthesis [see ✎ p. 722 box, Fig. 32.2].

2. Gram-positive organisms [see ✎ pp. 718, 684].

3. Acetylated metabolites of the **sulphonamides** could otherwise precipitate in the kidney tubules causing crystalluria and damage [see ✎ p. 722].

4. In the context of antibacterial agents the answer is **trimethoprim** but the statement is true for most chemotherapeutic folate antagonists [see ✎ Fig. 37.1].

5. (i) Benzylpenicillin and congeners, lactamase-resistant; (ii) broad-spectrum (and non-β-lactamase resistant); (iii) extended-spectrum with antipseudomonal activity; (iv) reversed-spectrum [see ✎ p. 729 box, Table 37.2].

6. **Benzylpenicillin** is active against most Gram-positive cocci and some Gram-negative bacteria [see ✎ p. 726].

7. Some examples are:

   a. Broad-spectrum: **ampicillin, amoxycillin**. Also **pivampicillin, talampicillin, bacampicillin**.

   b. β-lactamase-resistant: **cloxacillin, flucloxacillin**.

   c. Antipseudomonal: **carbenicillin, ticarcillin, azlocillin**.

   [See ✎ Table 37.2.]

8. **Penicillin** first binds to special binding proteins, then inhibits the transpeptidation enzyme that cross-links the peptide chains attached to the peptidoglycan backbone [see ✎ Fig. 35.3]. The final bactericidal event is inactivation of an inhibitor of the autolytic enzymes in the cell wall [see ✎ p. 724].

9. 'Bacteriostatic' means: 'stops growth by interfering with the metabolism of a bacterium without killing it'. 'Bactericidal' means: 'kills the bacterium' [see ✎ p. 722].

10. Bacteriostatic drugs include **sulphonamides, trimethoprim**. Bactericidal drugs include **all β-lactam antibiotics, aminoglycosides, polymixins**. Some drugs may be either bactericidal or bacteriostatic depending on the organism or the concentration of drug, e.g. **chloramphenicol, erythromycin, nalidixic acid, vancomycin, isoniazid**.

11. The production of β-lactamases; a reduction in the permeability of the outer membrane (Gram-negative organisms); modified penicillin-binding sites [see ✎ pp. 724–726].

12. **a.** Staphylococci; **b.** β-lactamase production; **c. clavulanic acid**; **d.** as a suicide inhibitor of β-lactamase [see ✎ pp. 724–726, Fig. 37.3].

13. Only when the meninges are inflamed [see ✎ p. 727].

14. Given by injection; $t_{1/2}$ 30 min after i.m. injection [see ✎ Table 37.2].

15. They are usually described in terms of generations: the 1st generation (e.g. **cephradine**) begat the 2nd generation (e.g. **cefachlor, cefuroxime**), which begat the 3rd generation (e.g. **cefotaxime**) ……… [see ✎ Table 37.3].

16. **Ceftazidime** (also **cefsoludin**) [see ✎ Table 37.3].

17. The carbapenem, **imipenem** [see ✎ p. 729 box].

18. The monobactam, **aztreonam** [see ✎ Fig. 37.3, p. 729 box].

19. Hypersensitivity reactions [see ✎ p. 727].

20. **Chloramphenicol** [see ✎ p. 732].

21. They all inhibit bacterial protein synthesis [see ✎ Fig. 35.4, p. 735 box].

22. **Chloramphenicol** [see ✎ p. 735 box].

PART

1

23. **Tetracyclines** [see 📖 p. 735 box].

24. The **aminoglycosides** [see 📖 p. 735 box].

25. First-line: **isoniazid**, **rifampicin**, **ethambutol**, **pyrazinamide**. Second-line: **capreomycin**, **cycloserine**, **streptomycin** [see 📖 p. 741 box]. (Streptomycin is used now in the UK mainly for resistant organisms.)

26. **a.** They inhibit topoisomerase II.

   b. Some examples are: **nalidixic acid**, **cinoxacin**, **norfloxacin**, **ciprofloxacin** [see 📖 Figs 37.7, 35.6, p. 735].

27. It may inhibit folate synthesis [see p. 742 box].

28. For tuberculosis (a first-line drug), and for tuberculoid leprosy [see 📖 pp. 741 box, 742 box].

29. **Ciprofloxacin** has a wide antibacterial spectrum being especially active against Gram-negative bacteria [see 📖 p. 737 box].

30. It would be best to steer clear of **gentamicin** which has ototoxicity that could potentiate any latent **frusemide**-mediated ototoxicity [see 📖 pp. 379, 733, 735 box].

31. **Ciprofloxacin**.

32. **A.** False; **tetracyclines** chelate calcium and are deposited in growing bones and teeth [see 📖 p. 735 box].

   B. False; they are broad-spectrum antibiotics [see 📖 p. 735 box].

   C. False; **vancomycin** is bactericidal but it acts by interfering with cell wall synthesis; the **polymixins** disrupt cell membranes by an interaction with phospholipids [see 📖 p. 738 box, Fig. 35.3].

   D. False; elimination is renal (remember the first clinical test of penicillin, in which it was extracted from the urine and used again—and again and again?) but it is eliminated by tubular secretion [see 📖 p. 727].

E. True [see 📖 p. 733].

F. True [see 📖 p. 732].

G. False; this is true of **clavulanic acid**; **cilastatin** is used with **imipenem** to inhibit the proximal tubule dehydropeptidase which breaks down imipenem, resulting in low urinary concentration of the antibacterial agent [see 📖 pp. 729, 726].

38

Antiviral drugs

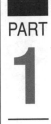

BACKGROUND INFORMATION

Viruses consist essentially of nucleic acid in a protein coat. Having no metabolic machinery of their own, they have to use the metabolic processes of the host cell, which they enter and infect. DNA viruses have to enter the host cell nucleus to direct the generation of new viruses. RNA viruses direct the generation of copies of themselves without involving the host cell nuclear material. RNA retroviruses (e.g. the AIDS virus) have an enzyme, reverse transcriptase, which makes a DNA copy of the viral RNA; this DNA copy is integrated into the host genome and directs the generation of new viral particles.

Because a virus virtually (in some cases, actually) becomes part of its host cell, selective chemotherapy is difficult. A degree of selectivity can be achieved by:

- agents which localise within infected cells because they are activated by the virus
- agents which inhibit specific viral enzymes.

The drugs available are:
Agents which inhibit attachment to or penetration of host cells: e.g. **amantadine**, γ-**globulin**
Agents which inhibit nucleic acid synthesis: e.g. **vidarabine**, **tribavirin**, **acyclovir**, **foscarnet** (phosphonoformate), **zidovudine**, **idoxuridine**, **ganciclovir**, **didanosine**, **zalcitabine**
Immunomodulators: e.g. **interferons**, **inosine**.

QUESTIONS

1. Name two antiviral drugs which may be effective against herpes viruses, e.g. herpes simplex, varicella-zoster which causes shingles.

2. What antiviral drugs may be effective against cytomegalovirus?

   (Cytomegalovirus is a type of herpes virus which can cause opportunistic infections of the foetus, also hepatitis or a type of glandular fever postnatally, and generalised infection in immunocompromised patients.)

3. What antiviral drugs may be effective against the respiratory syncytial virus? (This virus can cause colds, but its importance lies in the fact that it can cause bronchiolitis and pneumonia in infants. The main cold-causing viruses are rhinoviruses.)

4. The .... receptor in the host may function as a receptor/binding site for the rabies virus.

5. **a.** What is the mechanism of action of the anti-AIDS agent, **zidovudine**?

   b. How is it given?

6. What antiviral agent might be effective in Lassa fever—an arenavirus infection with high mortality?

7. Indicate which of the following statements are true and which false. If you think a statement is false, explain why.

   A. Acyclovir is only fully functional in infected cells because it needs to be phosphorylated by viral thymidine kinase.

   B. Ganciclovir is inactive until phosphorylated; this can be accomplished by either host or viral kinases.

   C. The mechanism of action of **acyclovir** triphosphate is by specific inhibition of viral RNA-polymerase.

   D. Idoxuridine is given orally in treatment of varicella-zoster (shingles).

   E. Foscarnet (phosphonoformate) inhibits viral DNA polymerase by binding

127

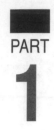

to the pyrophosphate binding site on viral DNA.

F. The β-adrenoceptor may function as a 'receptor' for the AIDS virus.

G. There is evidence that **tribavirin** can interfere with synthesis of viral mRNA.

H. Didanosine is used as an anti-AIDS agent.

I. Amantadine has been relatively effective in preventing some types of influenza.

J. Interferons act by inhibiting viral mRNA.

K. α-**interferon** is used to treat hepatitis B infection.

L. Acyclovir has proved effective in the treatment of herpes zoster (shingles) in immunocompromised patients.

M. Zalcitabine inhibits attachment of virus to cells and is used against influenza A.

ANSWERS

1. **Acyclovir** (the drug of choice), **idoxuridine**, **bromovinyldeoxyuridine**, **vidarabine**. (Foscarnet is active but too toxic) [see 📖 pp. 747, 749].

2. **Ganciclovir** (toxic [see 7B below], used only in very severe infections in immunocompromised patients), **foscarnet** (used for cytomegalovirus infections of the retina in AIDS patients) [see 📖 pp. 748, 749].

3. **Tribavirin**, in aerosol form [see 📖 p. 749].

4. Acetylcholine receptor on skeletal muscle [see 📖 Table 38.1].

5. **a.** It inhibits viral reverse transcriptase.

   b. Orally or i.v. [see 📖 p. 750].

6. Tribavirin [see 📖 p. 749].

7. **A.** True [see 📖 p. 748].

B. True; it is therefore more toxic to host cells than **acyclovir**, and can cause bone marrow depression, CNS disturbances, GIT upsets.

C. False; true for viral DNA-polymerase [see 📖 p. 748].

D. False; it is only ever used topically [see 📖 p. 749].

E. True [see 📖 p. 749].

F. False; the β-adrenoceptor is a binding site for the infantile diarrhoea virus. A 'receptor' for the AIDS virus is the CD_4 (T_4) molecule on T lymphocytes [see 📖 Table 38.1].

G. True [see 📖 p. 753 box].

H. True [see 📖 p. 751].

I. True [see 📖 p. 751].

J . False; they induce host cell enzymes which inhibit viral mRNA [see 📖 p. 753 box].

K. True [see 📖 p. 753].

L. True [see 📖 p. 749 box].

M. False; it is a reverse transcriptase inhibitor used with zidovudine in AIDS.

39

Antifungal drugs

BACKGROUND INFORMATION

Fungi can cause both superficial infections (of skin, hair, nails, mucous membranes) and infections of deeper tissues and organs. The commonest superficial infections are due to *Tinea* organisms, e.g. ringworm, athlete's foot. Oral candidiasis (thrush) may occur after inhaled glucocorticoids, broad-spectrum antibiotics or cytotoxic drugs. The commonest systemic fungal infection is systemic candidiasis. Opportunistic infections are increasing in incidence, especially in individuals with compromised immune systems, AIDS patients in particular.

The drugs used clinically are:
- Antifungal antibiotics, e.g. **amphotericin, nystatin, griseofulvin**.
- Synthetic antifungal agents, e.g. **fluconazole, itraconazole, miconazole, flucytosine**.

QUESTIONS

1. What is the mechanism of action of **amphotericin**?

2. .... is fungistatic and its mechanism of action involves an interaction with fungal microtubules and thus interference with mitosis.

3. What is the mechanism of action of the **azoles**?

4. A drug used topically to treat athlete's foot is ....?

5. What therapy is effective for oral candidiasis (thrush)?

6. Indicate which **antifungal azoles** can be given orally, and which can be given intrathecally?

7. The antifungal agent **a.** .... in high doses can cause gynaecomastia in males because **b.** ....

8. **a.** What is the mechanism of action of **flucytosine**?

   b. How is it given?

9. **Amphotericin** enhances the antifungal effect of ....

10. Indicate whether the following statements are true or false. If you think a statement is false, explain why.

    A. Ketoconazole, given orally, is the drug of choice for athlete's foot.

    B. Oral fluconazole can be used in the treatment of vaginal candidiasis.

    C. Flucytosine is mainly active against yeast infections.

    D. Nystatin is not absorbed from the GIT and is given parenterally.

    E. Griseofulvin, applied topically, is an effective treatment for fungal infections of the skin.

    F. A treatment for cryptococcol meningitis is intravenous **fluconazole**.

    G. Flucytosine acts by selectively binding to fungal cell membranes and interfering with permeability and transport functions.

ANSWERS

1. It disrupts the organisation of the membrane of fungal cells [see 📖 p. 756].

2. **Griseofulvin** [see 📖 p. 758].

3. **Azoles** inhibit the biosynthesis of ergosterol [see 📖 p. 759].

4. A topical **azole** [see 📖 Table 39.1].

5. Topical **nystatin** [see 📖 Table 39.1].

6. Orally: **fluconazole** (also i.v.), **itraconazole**, **miconazole** (for GIT infection). Intrathecal: **miconazole** [see 📖 pp. 759–760].

7. **a.** **Ketoconazole**; **b.** it inhibits steroidogenesis [see 📖 p. 759].

8. **a.** It is converted by a fungal enzyme to 5-fluorouracil, which inhibits thymidylate synthetase.

   b. Orally [see 📖 p. 758].

9. **Flucytosine** [see 📖 Table 39.1, p. 757].

10. **A.** False; **ketoconazole** can cause serious, sometimes fatal, liver toxicity; it is not used for superficial fungal infections such as athlete's foot. Topical azoles (**clotrimazole, econazole**) are the drugs used [see 📖 Table 39.1, pp. 759–760 and Answer 4 above].

    B. True [see 📖 Table 39.1].

    C. True; it is used for systemic yeast infections. Unwanted effects are not common but, if therapy is prolonged, monitoring of the blood count is advisable [see 📖 Table 39.1, p. 759].

    D. False; **nystatin** indeed is not absorbed from the GIT, but it is too toxic to be given parenterally. It is given orally for fungal infections in the intestine, and used topically for fungal infections of the skin [see 📖 p. 758].

    E. False; **griseofulvin** is effective for fungal infections of the skin, but it is inactive if applied topically. It is given orally and is taken up by skin cells. It is used when topical application of other drugs has been unsuccessful [see 📖 p. 758].

    F. True [see 📖 p. 759].

    G. False; the statement is true for **amphotericin**. **Flucytosine** is converted to the antimetabolite, 5-fluorouracil, which inhibits DNA synthesis [see 📖 pp. 756, 758].

40

Antiprotozoal drugs

BACKGROUND INFORMATION

The main protozoa that produce disease in man are those causing malaria, amoebiasis, leishmaniasis, trypanosomiasis and trichomoniasis.

Malaria

Malaria is caused by various species of plasmodia. The female anopheline mosquito injects *sporozoites* which can develop in the liver cells into either:

- schizonts which divide and form *merozoites* (the pre-erythrocytic stage); the merozoites when liberated infect red blood cells, then grow and divide to form and release another batch of merozoites, causing fever; this constitutes the erythrocytic stage
- dormant *hypnozoites* which may later divide to give rise to merozoites (the exoerythrocytic stage).

The main malarial parasites causing fever every third day (tertian malaria) are *Plasmodium vivax* which causes benign tertian malaria, and *Plasmodium falciparum* which causes malignant tertian malaria and which (unlike *Plasmodium vivax*) does not give rise to hypnozoites and thus has no exoerythrocytic stage. Some merozoites develop into male or female gametocytes which, when ingested by a mosquito, give rise to further stages of the parasite's lifecycle within the insect.

Antimalarial drugs are used mainly either (i) to treat the acute attack of malaria, acting on the erythrocytic stage (**chloroquine, quinine** with **pyrimethamine** with **sulphadoxine, halofantrine**) or (ii) for chemoprophylaxis (**chloroquine**, with or without **proguanil**), preventing an attack by killing the merozoites as they emerge from the liver before they can start the erythrocytic cycle. Some drugs (e.g. **primaquine**) can effect (iii) radical cure by acting on hypnozoites in the liver. (Note *P. falciparum* has no hypnozoite stage and can be cured by drugs which act on the erythrocytic stage.) Some drugs (iv) act on gametocytes and prevent transmission by the mosquito, reducing the human reservoir.

Pneumocystis carinii
A ?protozoon/?fungus that causes opportunistic pneumonia in AIDS patients.

Drugs used include **co-trimoxazole**.

Amoebiasis
Amoebiasis is due to infection with *Entamoeba histolytica* which invades the intestinal wall (and, rarely, the liver) and causes dysentery.

Drugs used: metronidazole, diloxanide.

Leishmaniasis
Leishmaniasis can occur as a skin infection or as an infection of the viscera. It is transmitted by blood-sucking flies.

Drugs used: metronidazole, sodium stibogluconate.

Trypanosomiasis
Two trypanosome species affect the CNS causing sleeping sickness, and another affects other internal organs causing Chagas' disease.

Drugs used: suramin for sleeping sickness, **pentamidine** for Chagas' disease.

Trichomoniasis
Trichomoniasis organisms cause vaginitis in females and sometimes urethritis in males.

Drug used: metronidazole.

Toxoplasmosis
This is an animal (e.g. cat) protozoon that can infect humans.

Drugs used include **pyrimethamine-sulphadiazine**.

QUESTIONS

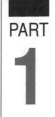

PART

1

1. **a.** What is the main drug used for *oral* treatment of the acute clinical attack of malaria?

   b. In what circumstances is it not used?

   c. What drugs are then used instead?

2. **a.** What is the main drug used for chemoprophylaxis of malaria?

   b. In what circumstances is it not used?

   c. What drugs are then used instead?

3. What drug is used when parenteral administration is necessary for the treatment of the acute clinical attack of malaria?

4. **a.** In the context of malaria, what is 'causal prophylaxis'?

   b. What are 'tissue schizonticides'?

   c. What are 'blood schizonticides'?

5. *Plasmodium* **a.** .... which causes a common form of malaria termed **b.** .... can cause multiple relapses giving repeated acute attacks, even if each attack is effectively treated with blood schizonticides, because **c.** ....

6. Which form of malaria has become resistant to **chloroquine** in many parts of the world?

7. What are the two main groups of drugs available for treatment of the acute clinical attack of malaria?

8. .... is a tissue schizonticidal drug which is effective against malarial parasites in the liver and can effect radical cure.

9. Name a combination of **a.** a drug which affects folate synthesis with **b.** a folate antagonist, which can be used (in combination) to treat the acute clinical attack and also for chemoprophylaxis. In what circumstances would this pair be used?

10. What are the main antimalarial actions of **chloroquine**?

11. What are the unwanted effects of **quinine**?

12. a. .... derived from a traditional Chinese remedy for malaria, has been effective in treating the acute clinical attack. Its main action is **b.** ....

13. In a patient with amoebiasis the causative organism may be present in two forms: **a.** ....; **b.** ....

14. What is the drug of choice for chronic intestinal amoebiasis in which cysts are present in the stools?

15. What drugs are used for hepatic amoebiasis?

16. Metronidazole is effective in a variety of infections. What are they?

17. Indicate whether the following statements are true or false. If you think a statement is false, explain why.

A. Proguanil has a t₁/₂ of 4 days and effective antimalarial plasma concentrations may last for 2 weeks.

B. Mefloquine can be used to treat the acute clinical attack of malaria caused by chloroquine-resistant *P. falciparum.*

C. Quinine is the drug used if parenteral therapy is required for the acute clinical attack of malaria.

D. Primaquine is used for radical cure of *P. vivax* malaria because it kills the sporozoites injected by the mosquito.

E. A severe but rare unwanted effect of therapy with **chloroquine** is blackwater fever.

F. Pyrimethamine and **proguanil** are used in combination because they inhibit the folate metabolism of the malarial parasite at different points.

G. Halofantrine is an amoebicide.

H. Diloxanide furoate has to be absorbed in order to exert anti-amoebiasis action.

I. Stibogluconate is the drug of choice for *Leishmania* infections of the viscera.

18. Indicate which of the following are true.

a. The main drug(s) used for the acute clinical attack of falciparum malaria in an area where plasmodia have not developed resistance to antimalarial drugs is/are:

A. Suramin   **B. Metronidazole**
C. Chloroquine   **D. Quinine.**

b. Drug(s) effective against the non-invasive form of the organism which causes amoebiasis are:

A. Diloxanide furoate B. Emetine
C. Pentamidine   **D. Chloroquine**
E. Pyrimethamine.

c. Drug(s) which can be effective in hepatic amoebiasis are:

A. Pyrimethamine   **B. Primaquine**
C. Chloroquine   **D. Stibogluconate**
E. Metronidazole.

ANSWERS

1. a. Chloroquine. b. Chloroquine-resistant malaria. **c.** Various regimes, e.g. **quinine** with either **pyrimethamine–sulpha-doxine** or **tetracycline**, or **mefloquine** alone [see 🔖 Table 40.1].

2. a. Chloroquine. b. It is not used by itself in choroquine-resistant malaria. **c.** Various regimes, e.g. **chloroquine** plus **pyrimethamine–dapsone**; or **chloroquine** plus **proguanil**; or **chloroquine** plus **doxycycline**; or **mefloquine** [see 🔖 Table 40.1].

3. Quinine [see 🔖 Table 40.1].

4. a. Another name for chemoprophylaxis.

b. Drugs affecting the malaria parasites within the liver [see 🔖 p. 765, where the term is confined to drugs acting on liver hypnozoites to produce radical cure. Some American textbooks extend the term to describe drugs used for chemoprophylaxis, some do not].

c. Drugs effective against the parasites in the blood and therefore used to treat the acute attack [see 🔖 Fig. 40.1].

5. **a.** *vivax;* **b.** benign tertian malaria;
c. hypnozoites are likely to be lurking in the liver [see 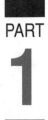 pp. 763, 763 box, Fig. 40.1].

6. Falciparum malaria [see 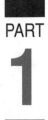 Fig. 40.2, Table 40.1].

7. (i) The quinoline-methanols and (ii) drugs acting on the synthesis and/or action of folate [see 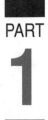 p. 764].

8. **Primaquine** [see 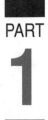 p. 769 box].

9. One example is **a. sulphadoxine** with **b. pyrimethamine**. The combination is used when dealing with chloroquine-resistant plasmodia (but see Answer 2 above) [see also 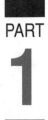 p. 769].

10. **Chloroquine** is:

    (i) a potent blood schizonticide and therefore used to treat the acute clinical attack (i.e. for suppressive or clinical cure);

    (ii) an effective agent for radical cure of *P. falciparum* since this parasite has no hypnozoite forms;

    (iii) an effective chemoprophylactic agent.

    Note these actions are only effective if the organism is not chloroquine-resistant [see 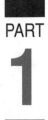 Fig. 40.2].

11. GIT upsets, tinnitus, blurred vision; with large doses, CNS and CVS disturbances [see 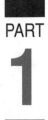 p. 767].

12. **a. Artemisinin; b.** as a fast-acting blood schizonticide [see 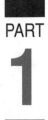 p. 771].

13. **a.** Cysts; **b.** trophozoites—the invasive form [see 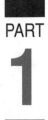 p. 772 box].

14. **Diloxanide furoate** [see 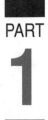 p. 772 box].

15. **Metronidazole** followed by **diloxanide** [see 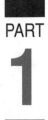 p. 772].

16. It is the drug of choice for invasive amoebic dysentery and amoebic hepatitis, for skin infections with *Leishmania* organisms, for trichomonas vaginitis and for *Giardia lamblia* infections. It is also effective against some Gram-negative bacilli, e.g. *Bacteroides, Clostridia* and some streptococci [see 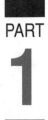 pp. 738, 772, 773, Table 37.1].

17. **A.** False; this statement is true for **pyrimethamine;** with **proguanil** the plasma concentration falls to zero in 24 hours [see 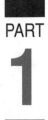 p. 769].

    B. True; it is also used combined with **pyrimethamine–sulphadoxine** [see 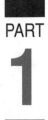 Table 40.1].

    C. True; used as the dihydrochloride or gluconate [see 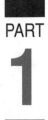 Table 40.1].

    D. False; nothing presently available kills the injected sporozoites. **Primaquine** is, however, used for radical cure [see 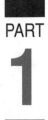 p. 769 box].

    E. False; this applies to **quinine** [see 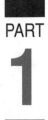 p. 767].

    F. False; the two drugs are both **folate antagonists. Proguanil** can be used alone; **pyrimethamine** is only used in combination with a **sulphonamide** or with **dapsone** [see 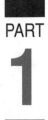 Fig. 40.4, Table 40.1, pp. 769, 769 box].

    G. False; it is a blood schizonticidal agent used to treat the clinical attack of chloroquine-resistant falciparum malaria [see 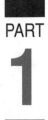 pp. 767, 769 box, 770 clinical box].

    H. False; it is the unabsorbed moiety in the GIT that is amoebicidal [see 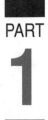 p. 772 box].

    I. True [see 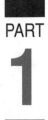 p. 773 box].

18. **a.** Only C is correct [see 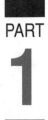 Table 40.1].

    b. Only A is correct [see 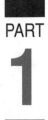 p. 772 box].

    c. E is correct. **Metronidazole** is the drug of choice [see 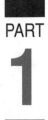 p. 772 box].

PART

1

41

Anthelminthic drugs

BACKGROUND INFORMATION

Some helminths (worms) infest the gastro-intestinal tract, e.g. tapeworms, roundworms; others infest the tissues of the body, e.g. bilharzia-causing flukes, tissue roundworms, hydatid tapeworms.

Drugs used clinically: piperazine, mebendazole, thiabendazole, pyrantel, niclosamide, praziquantel, oxamniquine, metriphonate, diethylcarbamazine.

QUESTIONS

1. Name two drugs effective in common roundworm infections.

2. **a.** .... causes paralysis of the common roundworm; it reversibly inhibits the worm's neuromuscular transmission in a GABA-like fashion.

   b. .... has both nicotinic-like and anticholinesterase actions resulting in spasm followed by paralysis.

   c. .... a potent antifilarial agent, probably acts by augmenting the action of GABA at the worm's neuromuscular junction.

3. Which is the drug of choice for the British threadworm and which for the American threadworm?

4. Why is the use of a purgative recommended after the use of **niclosamide** for the pork tapeworm?

5. Name two **benzimidazole anthelminthics** and describe the mode of action of these compounds.

CHAPTER 41

6. .... is a new broad-spectrum anthelminthic of low toxicity; it is the drug of choice for all schistosomes (worms causing bilharzia) and for cysticercosis (cysts of the pork tapeworm in the tissues).

7. Why might it be counterproductive to use **piperazine** and **pyrantel** simultaneously to treat roundworm?

8. **a.** .... an organophosphate anticholinesterase effective against *Schistosoma haematobium* is a pro-drug giving rise, spontaneously, in vivo, to the active compound **b.** ....

9. A drug with antifilarial activity is ....

10. What is the mechanism of action of **praziquantel**?

11. Which anthelminthics must be given parenterally for action against worms which live in the tissues of the host?

ANSWERS

1. Examples are: **levamisole**, **pyrantel**, **mebendazole**, **piperazine** [see 📖 Table 41.1].

2. **a. Piperazine**; **b. pyrantel**; **c. ivermectin** [see 📖 pp. 779, 781].

3. **Mebendazole** or **pyrantel** in the UK, **thiabendazole** in the USA. This is not binational perversity; the name is given to two quite different animals on either side of the Atlantic [see 📖 Table 41.1].

4. To remove dead worms before ova are released. The use of an anti-emetic would be an additional wise precaution [see 📖 p. 779].

5. **Thiabendazole**, **mebendazole**, albendazole. They inhibit helminth microtubular function [see 📖 p. 777].

6. **Praziquantel**; not marketed in the UK [see 📖 p. 779].

7. These two agents might well cancel out each other's actions on the helminth

neuromuscular junction; **piperazine** hyperpolarises, **pyrantel** depolarises [see 📖 p. 779].

8. **a. Metriphonate**; **b. dichlorvos** [see 📖 p. 780].

9. Some examples are: **diethylcarbamazine**, **albendazole**, **ivermectin** [see 📖 Table 41.1].

10. It acts on the plasma membrane of helminth cells causing increased Ca^{2+} permeability [see 📖 p. 779].

11. All the drugs listed in this chapter are given by mouth. **Suramin**, a trypanosomicidal drug, is used i.v. subsequent to **invermectin** for infestation with *Onchocera volvulus* in some treatment regimes; it is very toxic.

42

Individual variation and drug interaction

BACKGROUND INFORMATION

That cells, or tissues, or individual animals or humans vary in response to a chemical stimulus is a fact of life. This biological variation bedevils pharmacological experiments and clinical practice. Variation in the effects of a drug between individuals or in one individual at different times can be due either to different concentrations of the drug reaching the site of action or to different responses to the same concentration. The former is pharmacokinetic variation, the latter pharmacodynamic. Age, disease states, drug interactions and genetic factors are all important in the variation in response to drugs. Age can alter both renal function and drug metabolism and thus the effective concentration of the drug or its effects. Idiosyncratic reactions to drugs, which usually only occur in a small number of individuals, can be the basis of harmful reactions; genetic factors are often involved in such reactions. Diseases, especially of the major drug eliminating organs, the liver and kidney, may obviously have important effects on the concentration of drug in the body. Finally, drug interactions, which can be pharmacodynamic and pharmacokinetic, can contribute to variation. The former are predictable from the effects of the interacting drugs, the latter can involve variation in absorption, metabolism and excretion.

QUESTIONS

Many of the questions on this topic are in Part 2 since they are best dealt with when the reader has more knowledge of the actions on individual drugs.

1. **a.** What are the main types of variability?

PART

1

b. What are the main causes of variability?

2. In the neonate or the elderly, is renal excretion increased or decreased?

3. On the basis of the answers to Question 2, what would happen to the plasma half-life of a drug in a neonate, or in a woman of 75?

4. Why can **chloramphenicol** and **morphine** cause problems in premature babies?

5. Why can **diazepam** be more effective, or cause more side effects in the elderly?

6. Give an example of a drug where plasma cholinesterase activity can be so inefficient, due to genetic variation, that what is normally a few minutes' duration of action becomes several hours.

7. **a.** What is the main type of drug interaction involving effects on distribution?

   b. What are the consequences of this type of interaction?

8. Give two examples of drugs which induce drug-metabolising enzymes.

9. How might a drug with effects on the heart affect the response to another drug?

10. How might drugs which affect renal function alter the response to other drugs?

ANSWERS

1 . **a.** Pharmacokinetic, pharmacodynamic and idiosyncratic.

   b. Age (very young or old), genetic factors, drug interactions and pathological or physiological states [see 📖 p. 785 box].

2. Renal excretion is reduced in both; it is 20% of the adult value at birth but it rapidly reaches adult levels by 1 week. At the age of 75, renal function is about half that of a 20-year-old [see 📖 p. 786].

3. It will increase, with all the repercussions implied by this fact [see 📖 p. 786, Table 42.1].

4. In these babies, the conjugating enzymes in the liver are immature so that biotransformation is slowed and accumulation of the drugs can thus occur [see 📖 pp. 786–787].

5. The metabolism of diazepam occurs at a slower rate in the elderly, leading to a longer plasma half-life and potentially higher plasma concentrations of the drug. In addition, at the same plasma concentration as in a younger subject, **benzodiazepines** produce more of an effect in the elderly [see 📖 p. 787, Fig. 42.2].

6. **Suxamethonium**, the neuromuscular blocker [see 📖 p. 788 and Fig. 42.4].

7. **a.** Competition for plasma protein binding. A large proportion of the drug being bound to plasma protein is a prerequisite for this type of interaction to be significant, as is a high dose of the displacing drug.

   b. Complex. The free concentration of the displaced drug rises, but metabolism and excretion can then increase so that the total plasma concentration may decrease.

8. Some examples are: **barbiturates**, **phenytoin**, **alcohol**, **carbamazepine**, **rifampicin** [see 📖 p. 793, Table 42.2].

9. A drug which decreases cardiac output and thereby hepatic blood flow (e.g. **propranolol**) may reduce metabolism of agents which undergo extensive metabolism in the liver (e.g. **lignocaine**).

10. **Probenecid** reduces tubular secretion, so prolonging the action of penicillin and indomethacin. **Sulphonamides**, **aspirin**, and **thiazides** have a similar effect [see 📖 p. 795, Table 42.4]. **Diuretics** per se increase the excretion of other drugs.

43

Harmful effects of drugs

BACKGROUND INFORMATION

Some harmful effects of drugs are directly related to the main pharmacological actions of the agent (e.g. bleeding with **anticoagulants**, coma with **hypnotics**). Other harmful effects may be totally unrelated to the pharmacological actions (e.g. liver damage with **paracetamol**.) The phenomena in this second category are usually due to reactive metabolites and are often more serious than those in the first category. The mechanisms of cell damage and cell death may involve non-covalent and/or covalent interactions with target molecules.

Non-covalent interactions include:

- lipid peroxidation
- generation of cytotoxic oxygen radicals
- reactions causing depletion of glutathione
- modification of SH groups on key enzymes and structural proteins.

Covalent interaction can involve the macro-molecules of the cell. These interactions may result in the production of an immunogen (and subsequent allergic reactions), or, if DNA is the target, in carcinogenesis or teratogenesis.

QUESTIONS

1. How might reactive metabolites, produced when a drug is metabolised, cause cell damage by interacting with polyunsaturated lipids?

2. What might be the basis for the kidney damage which can result from therapy with **cyclosporin**?

3. Define: primary carcinogen, secondary carcinogen, promoter, co-carcinogen.

4. At what stage in the life of a female would mutagenesis of her germ cells be most likely to occur on exposure to a mutagen?

5. Indicate whether the following statements are true or false. If you think a statement is false, explain why.

   A. About three-quarters of the deaths caused by drug-induced anaphylactic shock are due to **penicillin**.

   B. In the Ames test for secondary carcinogens, the drug to be tested is added to a culture of mutant bacteria to determine whether it can directly cause a back mutation (i.e. reversion from mutant to wild type).

   C. Teratogenic drugs are most likely to cause gross malformation in the foetus if given in the fourth month of pregnancy.

   D. The main toxic effect which may result from the non-covalent interactions which can occur with repeated use of **halothane** in high concentration is acute papillary necrosis in the kidney.

   E. Phorbol esters are powerful secondary carcinogens.

ANSWERS

1. Reactive metabolite radicals could initiate lipid peroxidation. The lipid peroxyradicals (ROO˙) could then produce lipid hydroperoxides (ROOH) which could then produce further lipid peroxyradicals. This chain reaction could eventually affect much of the membrane lipid. Cell damage would result from alterations of membrane permeability or from reactions of the products of lipid peroxidation with proteins [see 📖 pp. 800–801].

2. It causes changes in renal vascular dynamics, possibly by decreasing the production of the vasodilator prostaglandins which would normally compensate for angiotensin-II-mediated vasoconstriction.

137

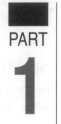

3. A primary carcinogen causes mutations directly, a secondary carcinogen only after conversion to active metabolites. Promoters and co-carcinogens are substances which, though not themselves carcinogenic, facilitate the development of cancer—promoters if given after the carcinogen; co-carcinogens if given with it [see 🖐 pp. 805–806].

4. While she is still an embryo in her mother's uterus, unlikely as this may seem [see 🖐 p. 805 box].

5. **A.** True [see 🖐 p. 812].

   B. False; primary carcinogens might directly cause mutation. Drugs which are secondary carcinogens need to be converted to the active metabolite; consequently a liver microsomal enzyme preparation must be included in the assay to generate the reactive metabolites [see 🖐 pp. 806, 807 box].

   C. False; teratogens cause gross malformations if given during the stage of organogenesis, i.e. between 17–60 days approximately. By the fourth month gross structural malformations are much less likely to occur [see 🖐 Table 43.5].

   D. False; it is liver damage [see 🖐 p. 802]. **Phenacetin** (now withdrawn) was the main culprit causing acute papillary necrosis, but other **NSAIDs** are reported to cause this occasionally.

   E. False. Phorbol esters have both promoter and co-carcinogen activity but are not themselves carcinogens [see 🖐 p. 806].

44

The pharmacology of smooth muscle

BACKGROUND INFORMATION

Many important pathological conditions involve disturbances of smooth muscle function, e.g. hypertension, bronchial asthma, gastrointestinal disorders, atony of the bladder, bile duct spasm. There are a host of mediators and drugs which act on smooth muscle. For all of these, the actions are well known; for many, the outline of the signal transduction mechanisms have been elucidated and, for most, the receptors have been extensively characterised and some have even been cloned. But surprisingly, the interest of many pharmacologists seems to stop at the receptor; surprising, since smooth muscle is one of the few tissues for which we now know most of the main steps leading from receptor stimulation to response. Smooth muscle is no longer a black box; we can delineate the pharmacological action of many agents virtually from their entry into the body through to the final response—contraction or relaxation of the relevant smooth muscle tissue.

Signal-transduction mechanisms in smooth muscle; or 'What's going on in there?'

Contraction. The transduction mechanism involves a rise in $[Ca^{2+}]_i$ which, via calmodulin, activates myosin-light-chain kinase. This phosphorylates light chains in the heads of the bipolar myosin filaments which allows the heads to pull on the actin filaments (Fig. 20); the heads then dissociate from the actin filaments and re-attach, and the power stroke is repeated, i.e. the heads 'walk' along the actin filaments, causing contraction of the muscle cell. The calcium which functions as internal messenger for contraction can be derived from the extracellular fluid or from internal calcium stores in the sarcoplasmic reticulum.

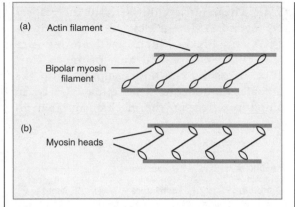

Fig. 20 Schematic diagram showing the mechanism of contraction in smooth muscle. The power stroke which converts (a) to (b) consists of a change in the conformation of the heads of the bipolar myosin filaments and involves phosphorylation of light chains in the individual myosin molecules which make up the myosin filament.

The concentration of calcium in the resting smooth muscle cell is about 100 nmol/l, and that in the extracellular fluid is about 2.5 mmol/l (i.e. approximately 25 000 times as much as the intracellular concentration). Stimulation of the relevant receptors increases intracellular Ca^{2+} by:

- activating ligand-operated ion channels, the resulting influx of Na^+ and Ca^{2+} causing membrane depolarisation which opens voltage-dependent Ca^{2+} channels [see Fig. 21]
- activating phospholipase C (PLC), via a G-protein; PLC hydrolyses PIP_2 to give both diacylglycerol (DAG) and inositol trisphosphate ($InsP_3$). $InsP_3$ acts on a receptor in the sarcoplasmic reticulum

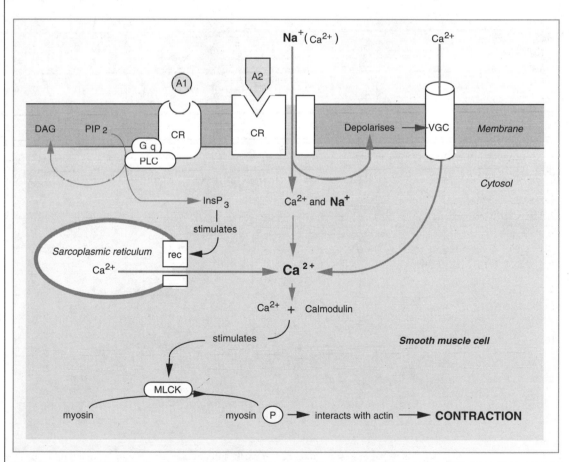

Fig. 21 The transduction mechanisms for contraction of smooth muscle. Calcium is the main internal messenger. CR = receptor causing contraction; A = agonists stimulating receptors causing contraction, some (A1) by activating receptors coupled to G-proteins, some (A2) by activating ligand-gated calcium channels (e.g. ATP); DAG = diacylglycerol; PLC = phospholipase C; Gq = G-protein which activates PLC; MLCK = myosin-light-chain kinase; VGC = voltage-gated calcium channel; PIP_2 = phosphatidylinositol bisphosphate; Rec = receptor in sarcoplasmic reticulum; $InsP_3$ = inositol trisphosphate.

(SR) opening a calcium channel in the SR, allowing efflux of stored Ca^{2+} [see Fig. 21]
• activating putative receptor-operated Ca^{2+} channels.

Relaxation. The transduction mechanism involves increases of cyclic AMP and cyclic GMP. These nucleotides activate the respective cyclic AMP and cyclic GMP kinases (PKA and PKG) which inactivate myosin-light-chain kinase and also promote Ca^{2+} efflux from the cell and re-uptake into the sarcoplasmic reticulum; there may also be an inhibitory effect on the mechanisms that in-

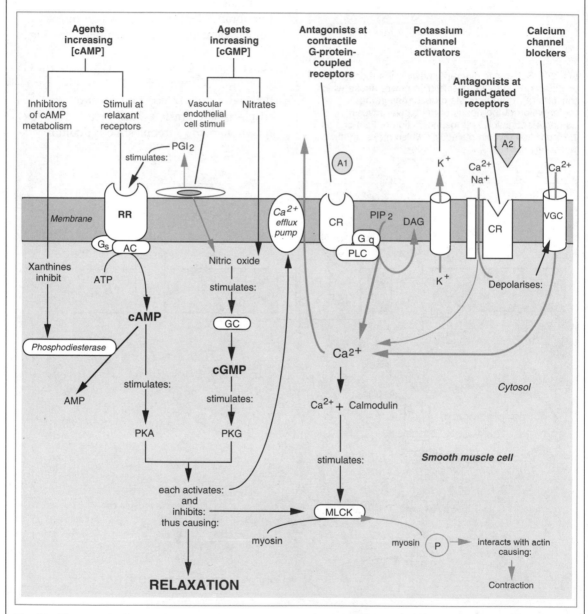

Fig. 22 The transduction mechanisms for relaxation in smooth muscle and the classes of drugs causing relaxation. RR = receptor causing relaxation; CR = receptor causing contraction; GC = guanylate cyclase; AC = adenylate cyclase; G_s = G-protein stimulating adenylate cyclase; PGI_2 = prostacyclin; PKA = cAMP-activated kinase; PKG = cGMP-activated kinase; MLCK = myosin-light-chain kinase; A = contractile agonist; VGC = voltage-gated calcium channel. Vascular endothelial cells release PGI_2 continuously and are also stimulated by some endogenous substances (e.g. acetylcholine, histamine) to release nitric oxide.

crease $[Ca^{2+}]_i$, e.g. inhibition of phospholipases C or D.

The increased opening of K^+ channels which results in efflux of K^+ and therefore hyperpolarisation and reduction of excitability, is another mechanism causing relaxation [see Fig. 22].

Mediators, transmitters and drugs can produce contraction of smooth muscle by acting either on receptors or on postreceptor mechanisms such as ion channels. They can produce relaxation by:

- activating receptors mediating relaxation
- affecting postreceptor transduction events for relaxation
- interfering with the receptors and transduction events involved in contractile responses.

A variety of different agents can influence the responses of smooth muscle, and their importance may differ in different tissues. Many drugs which affect smooth muscle function are important in clinical medicine.

In this chapter we will consider information on smooth muscle from the chapters on the circulation, the respiratory system, the uterus, the gastrointestinal tract, the sympathetic system and the parasympathetic system [all the mediators and drugs considered here are dealt with in most pharmacology textbooks; see ⬦ Chs 6, 7, 11, 13, 14, 17, 18, 19, 20, 21, 22].

QUESTIONS

1. Figure 21 shows, in schematic form, the transduction mechanisms for contraction of smooth muscle. List the drugs which cause contraction, by a direct action on smooth muscle, specifying the receptors on which they act in: **a.** blood vessels; **b.** bronchi; **c.** the GIT; **d.** the eye; **e.** the bladder; **f.** the myometrium. Specify the clinical significance (i.e. uses or pathological importance) of the drugs listed.

2. What pharmacological agents can cause contraction of smooth muscle by action on non-receptor mechanisms?

3. Figure 22 shows, in schematic form, the potential transduction mechanisms for relaxation of smooth muscle and the main classes of drugs inducing relaxation. List the individual drugs/mediators which can induce relaxation, specifying how they accomplish this and what the main clinical significance (i.e. therapeutic use or pathological importance) of their action is, on: **a.** vascular muscle; **b.** bronchial muscle; **c.** the GIT; **d.** the eye; **e.** the myometrium.

Note that additional mechanisms by which the cAMP/PKA system can produce relaxation have now been identified, viz. inhibition of PIP_2 hydrolysis, promotion of calcium re-uptake into the sarcoplasmic reticulum and activation of K^+ channels. These have not been included in Figure 22.

ANSWERS

1. Most pharmacological agents cause contraction by acting as agonists directly on receptors. Examples are given in Table 1.

2. Some dihydropyridines, e.g. BAYK 8644, promote the opening of voltage-operated Ca^{2+} channels [see ⬦ p. 298]. Potassium salts and Ca^{2+} ionophores cause depolarisation of the membrane. These agents are used as experimental tools.

3. Pharmacological agents can cause relaxation* by five major mechanisms [shown in Fig. 22] as follows:

- Increasing the concentration of cAMP, either by stimulating the receptors mediating relaxation or by inhibiting cAMP metabolism.

- Increasing the concentration of cGMP by giving rise to nitric oxide which activates guanylate cyclase. In vascular tissue, endothelial cells when

---

* Drugs causing relaxation of smooth muscle are particularly important clinically. Many work by interfering with contractile mechanisms.

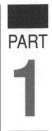

PART

1

Table 1 Agents causing contraction of smooth muscle

Tissue	Clinical significance
(a) Vascular smooth muscle	
α_1-receptors	
Noradrenaline	–
Adrenaline	*Uses*: anaphylactic shock; for vasoconstriction with local anaesthetics [see 📄 Table 7.4]
Methoxamine	*Use:* to counter hypotension during anaesthesia [see 📄 Table 7.4]
Phenylephrine	*Use:* nasal decongestant (some hypotensive states) [see 📄 Table 7.4]
Xylometazoline ⎫ Oxymetazoline ⎭	*Use:* nasal decongestant [see 📄 p. 162 box]
Dopamine	*Use:* infused for hypotensive shock [see 📄 Table 14.3]
Vasopressin, V_1-receptor agonist: felypressin	*Use*: vasoconstrictor adjunct to local anaesthetics [see 📄 Table 34.2]
Angiotensin II on angiotensin II receptors [see 📄 Fig. 14.5]	Involved in hypertension
Endothelin on endothelin receptors [see 📄 Table 14.3]	–
Adenosine on A_1-receptors in renal vasculature [see 📄 pp. 188–189]	–
5-HT on $5-HT_2$ receptors (constricts venules not arterioles) [see 📄 Fig. 8.3]	–
Thromboxane A_2 on TP-receptors [see 📄 p. 234 box]	–
LTD_4 on LTD_4 receptors (constricts only small coronary vessels) [see 📄 p. 237 box]	(Involved in coronary insufficiency)
(b) Bronchial muscle	
Adenosine on A_1-receptors [see 📄 pp. 188–189]	
Muscarinic M_3-receptors Acetylcholine, carbachol	Involved in reflex bronchoconstriction in bronchitis [see 📄 pp. 355 box, 360 box]
LTD_4 on leukotriene D_4-receptors	Mediator in asthma [see 📄 Fig. 17.3]
Histamine H_1-receptor agonists Histamine	Mediator in first phase of asthma [see 📄 Fig. 17.3]
2-methylhistamine	(Experimental tool)
β_2-receptor antagonists Propranolol	Can trigger bronchoconstriction in asthmatics by inhibiting the action of the endogenous adrenaline which would otherwise oppose the effect of inflammatory spasmogens [see 📄 p. 166]
(c) GIT muscle	Sometimes used for postoperative intestinal atony
Bethanechol on muscarinic M_3-receptors	Mediator of GIT inflammatory disorders? [see 📄 p. 234]
PGE_2 on EP_1- and EP_3-receptors	
α_1-adrenoceptor agonists on sphincter muscle	—
(d) Smooth muscle in the eye	

Muscarinic M_3-receptors on constrictor pupillae and ciliary muscle
    Pilocarpine
    Carbachol
	Use: glaucoma [see 📄 p. 128 box]

α_1-adrenoceptors on dilator pupillae Adrenaline [see 📄 Table 7.1]	

Table 1 *Continued*

Tissue	Clinical significance
(e) The bladder	
Bethanechol on muscarinic M_3-receptors [see 🖊 p. 126]	*Use:* in postoperative atony
(f) The myometrium	
Oxytocin on oxytocin receptors	*Use:* in postpartum haemorrhage; management of 3rd stage of labour [see 🖊 p. 472 box]
Ergometrine on α_1-receptors (and possibly 5-HT$_2$ receptors)	*Use:* in postpartum haemorrhage
Carboprost (15 methyl PGF$_{2\alpha}$) on FP-receptors	*Use:* in postpartum haemorrhage [see 🖊 p. 472 box)
PGE$_2$ and dinoprostone on EP$_3$-receptors	Involved in spasmodic dysmenorrhoea [see Prostaglandins in Ch. 22]
PGE$_{2\alpha}$ and dinoprost on FP-receptors	*Use*: therapeutic abortion [see 🖊 p. 472 box]
Histamine on H$_1$-receptors [see 🖊 Table 11.1a]	
Carbachol on M$_3$-receptors [see 🖊 Fig. 22.7, Table 6.1]	Experimental tools
Vasopressin on V$_1$-receptors [see 🖊 Fig. 2.7, Table 14.3]	

Table 2 Agents causing relaxation of smooth muscle

Tissue	Clinical significance
(a) Vascular smooth muscle	
Adrenaline on β-receptors [see 🖊 Table 7.1]	–
Dopamine on dopamine receptors (in mesenteric vessels) [see 🖊 p. 309]	–
5-HT on 5-HT$_2$ receptors in arterioles [see 🖊 Fig. 8.3]	–
Histamine on H$_1$- and H$_2$-receptors	
PGD$_2$ on DP-receptors	
PGE$_2$ on EP$_2$-receptors	
LTD$_4$ on LTD$_4$-receptors	Mediators of inflammation [see 🖊 Ch. 11]
PAF on PAF-receptors	
PGI$_2$ on IP-receptors	
Bradykinin on B$_2$-receptors (but most vasodilator effects are indirect)	
Antagonists at α_1-receptors	
Prazosin	*Use:* hypertension [see 🖊 Tables 7.4, 14.5]
Phenoxybenzamine / Phentolamine	*Use*: phaeochromocytoma [see 🖊 Table 7.4]
Ergotamine	*Use:* migraine [see 🖊 Table 7.4, p. 187 box]
Labetalol (antagonist also at β-receptors)	*Use:* hypertension [see 🖊 Table 7.4]
Antagonist at angiotensin II receptors Saralasin	*Potential use:* hypertension [see 🖊 Table 14.3, p. 316]
Calcium channel antagonists Nifedipine, diltiazem (affect mainly arteries)	*Use:* angina pectoris [see 🖊 p. 297 box]

Table 2 *Continued*

Tissue	Clinical significance
K+ channel openers	
Minoxidil, diazoxide	*Use:* hypertension [see 📖 Tables 14.3, 14.5]
Cromakalim, pinacidil	(*Potential use:* hypertension) [see 📖 Table 14.3]
Guanylate cyclase activators	
Nitrates (glyceryltrinitrate, isosorbide dinitrate, pentaerythritol tetranitrate)	*Use*: angina (also heart failure, biliary spasm) [see 📖 Tables 14.3, 13.3, Fig. 14.9, p. 312 box]
Sodium nitroprusside	*Use:* hypertensive crisis [see 📖 pp. 295 box, 312 box]
Nitric oxide (released by endothelium or generated from organic nitrate drugs) [see 📖 Fig. 14.1, Table 14.3, Ch. 10]	–
Peptides	
VIP (co-transmitter with ACh) [see 📖 Table 5.2]	–
Adenosine on A$_2$-receptors [see 📖 pp. 188–189]	–
PGI$_2$ on IP-receptors (released by endothelium stimulated by some vasodilators, e.g. bradykinin) [see 📖 pp. 241 box, 234]	–
(b) Bronchial muscle	
β$_2$-agonists	
Salbutamol, terbutaline	*Use:* asthma [see 📖 Fig. 17.3]
Adrenaline	*Use:* asthma (emergency) [see 📖 Table 7.4]
Phosphodiesterase inhibitors	*Use:* asthma [see 📖 p. 360 box]
Theophylline, aminophylline, enprofylline	
(c) The GIT	
Muscarinic M$_3$-receptor antagonists	*Use:* GIT disorders with smooth muscle spasm [see 📖 p. 129 box]
Pirenzipine	
PGE$_2$ on EP$_2$-receptors	–
PGD$_2$ pn DP-receptors	–
[see 📖 p. 233]	
(d) The smooth muscle in the eye	
Muscarinic M$_2$-receptor antagonists on constrictor pupillae [see 📖 p. 129 box]	
Tropicamide, homatropine cyclopentolate (also act on ciliary muscle)	*Use:* to produce mydriasis for examination of retina
Atropine	*Use*: iritis, eye surgery adjunct
(e) The myometrium	
β$_2$-receptor agonists	*Use:* to inhibit premature labour [see 📖 p. 470]
Salbutamol, terbutaline, ritodrine	
PGD$_2$ on DP-receptors [see 📖 p. 233]	–

stimulated by some mediators can release nitric oxide, or generate prostacyclin which stimulates an IP receptor that activates adenylate cyclase.

- Antagonising the action of agonists on the receptors mediating contraction.

- Activating K+ channels allowing efflux of K+ with resultant hyperpolarisation and subsequent relaxation.

- Blocking calcium channels.

PART 2

Questions

1. In a patient being treated with a cardiac glycoside, why might therapy with frusemide increase the incidence of toxic effects of the glycoside? How might this be prevented?

2. What is the main difference in the regulation of the secretion of the glucocorticoids as compared with that of the thyroid hormones—a difference which has a bearing on the use of drugs to stimulate the former and inhibit the latter? What drugs could be used in each case?

3. If a gardener inhales a large amount of an organophosphate insecticide spray, what might be the main effects? What would be the basis of the action?

4. Preparations of aspirin can be bought over the counter of all pharmacies and are even available in supermarkets and station bookstalls. Many people take aspirin for headache and for minor aches and pains. But if a patient is taking another pharmaceutical compound, the possibility of an interaction between aspirin and the prescribed drug exists. Name four drugs whose interaction with a *large* dose of aspirin could lead to significant clinical effects. Explain the mechanism of the interaction and outline the possible results.

5. One drug may reduce the effects of another by several different mechanisms [see 📖 Ch. 1]:

   a. chemical antagonism

   b. pharmacokinetic antagonism

   c. antagonism by receptor block which is:

   (i) reversible, competitive

   (ii) irreversible (non-equilibrium)

   d. block of receptor–effector linkage

   e. physiological antagonism.

   State which of the mechanisms listed above (if any) apply to:

   A. The decrease of the action of warfarin by phenobarbitone

   B. The effect of dimercaprol in poisoning by inorganic mercurial compounds

   C. The effect of nifedipine on noradrenaline-induced vasoconstriction

   D. The effect of salbutamol on histamine-induced bronchoconstriction

   E. The effect of phenoxybenzamine on noradrenaline-induced vasoconstriction

   F. The effect of trimetaphan on the stimulation of autonomic ganglia by acetylcholine

   G. The action of cimetidine on histamine-induced gastric secretion.

6. An elderly patient with rheumatoid arthritis (which has not responded to treatment with NSAIDs) experiences reasonable improvement in joint function after taking small daily doses of prednisolone for several months. Hoping for further improvement, she asks to be put on to a larger dose of steroid, requesting that she be given 6 months' supply to save repeat visits and promising that she will stop taking the tablets if she feels any ill effects. What drug therapy would you consider?

7. What potential problems might occur if a patient, who is taking **a.** cimetidine for a peptic ulcer, is given a course of **b.** warfarin for an episode of deep vein thrombosis, and who then also takes **c.** aspirin for a headache?

8. When a clot has formed after damage to normal blood vessels, serum plasminogen (P) is deposited on the fibrin strands and also on endothelial

cells; plasminogen activator (PA) is secreted by endothelial cells and may be bound to them. Interaction of P and PA gives rise to the fibrinolytic enzyme, plasmin. What factors in an atherosclerotic lesion may interfere with this process?

9. **a.** What is the transmitter at (i) autonomic ganglia, (ii) the postganglionic parasympathetic nerve terminal? What are the main receptors and transduction mechanisms involved in transmitter action at these sites? What drug groups can modify events at these sites and how do they work? Give examples of each group.

b. List the main subclasses of muscarinic receptors, indicating where they are located and what their transduction mechanisms are. Give examples of drugs used clinically which act on, or give rise to action on, muscarinic receptors:

in the GIT (specify uses);

in the urinary tract (specify uses);

in the eye (specify uses);

in the bronchi and bronchioles (specify uses);

for motion sickness (specify locus of action);

for Parkinson's disease (outline rationale for use).

Where possible indicate the receptors on which the agents act.

10. In a schematic diagram of the renal tubule such as that shown in Figure 23 indicate the following:

a. the areas where there is a high salt concentration in the interstitia, and the sites and mechanisms of action of the main hormones controlling active salt and water reabsorption

b. the sites of action of the main diuretics, with their mechanisms of action and principal characteristics

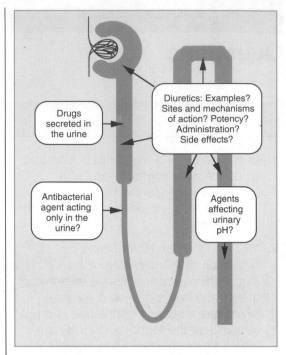

Fig. 23 Schematic diagram of renal tubule.

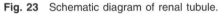

c. the site of active secretion of drugs into the tubule, with examples of agents secreted

d. examples of agents affecting urinary pH

e. an antibacterial agent which acts only in the urine.

11. The flow diagram, Figure 24, shows some of the factors which control blood pressure. Indicate the sites at which antihypertensive drugs could work and specify the receptors on which they act and/or their main mechanisms of action. (To answer this effectively you will probably need to sketch out the diagram on A4 paper.) Which are the drugs of first choice for treatment of hypertension? Which antihypertensive drugs are given parenterally?

12. A patient with chronic obstructive airways disease, who is obtaining considerable therapeutic benefit from a slow-release theophylline preparation, develops a serious gastroenteritis due to coliform organisms resistant to broad-spectrum penicillins, cephalosporins and

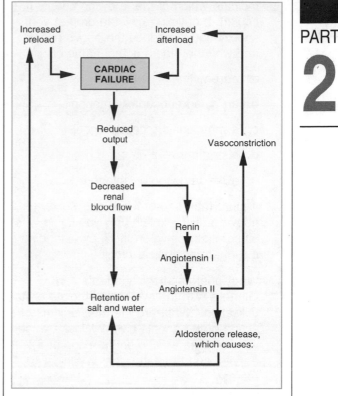

PART
2

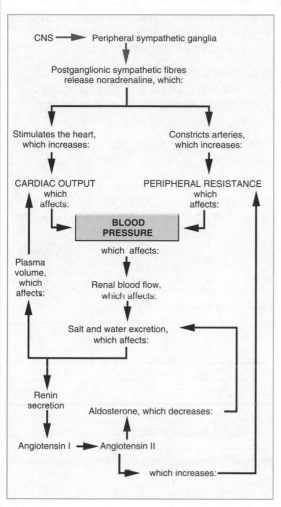

Fig. 24 Diagram of the main homeostatic mechanisms involved in the control of blood pressure.

Fig. 25 Diagram of the vicious circle of processes which may underlie cardiac failure.

such as might occur in a patient with myocardial infarction. The main therapeutic aims are: to improve contractility; to reduce afterload; and to optimise preload.

a. Indicate the sites of action of the drugs which could be used to accomplish these aims, giving examples of each group of agents. (You might find it useful to sketch out this diagram on A4 paper, before answering the question.)

b. Outline briefly the mechanism of action of the drugs cited.

aminoglycosides, but sensitive to ciprofloxacin and trimethoprim. Which of these would you choose (if you were the clinician) or recommend (if you were a pharmacologist who was asked for an opinion), and why?

13. What are the therapeutic uses of magnesium salts?

14. Name two drugs which act by forming covalent bonds with their target molecules?

15. The flow diagram in Figure 25 shows a simplified version of the vicious circle which underlies the pathogenesis of heart failure, with impaired contractility,

16. A drug, X, when tested experimentally for its pharmacological profile:

- reduces blood pressure after a bolus i.v. injection

- contracts the isolated guinea-pig ileum preparation

- causes bronchoconstriction.

149

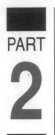

PART

2

Indicate which of the following agents it could be, outlining how the drug(s) you specify could produce the above effects and why the others do not fit the bill:

a. adrenaline

b. an α_1-adrenoceptor antagonist

c. a muscarinic receptor agonist

d. histamine

e. a β-adrenoceptor antagonist.

If more than one of these could give the above profile, explain how you could differentiate between them by extending the pharmacological profile.

17. What pharmacological agents can interfere with the synthesis of folate or its utilisation? What are the mechanisms of action of the agents given? What are the various uses which can be made of these agents, and of folate itself, in clinical therapy?

18. A patient being treated for hypertension develops red swollen joints in a big toe, such that anyone going near the toe causes an anxiety-based increase in pain.

a. Which drugs that might have been used to treat the hypertension could have produced this situation and what is the basis of the complaint?

b. What drugs could be used to treat the condition in the short term; in the long term?

Would you use NSAIDs for the pain, and if so which would you avoid and why?

19. Most pharmacology textbooks include a multitude of chemical formulae. It is clearly crucial for medicinal chemistry students and can be instructive for many pharmacology students to know the chemical structures of transmitters/ mediators/drugs. Name the structures shown in Figure 26 and give reasons why knowing them could aid your understanding of pharmacology.

20. How do the signal-transduction mechanisms for acetylcholine action on skeletal muscle differ from those for its action on GIT smooth muscle?

21. a. Name three endogenous peptides which are important in physiological/ pathological processes and for which competitive antagonists are known.

b. Specify conditions for which a peptide or peptide antagonist could be useful therapeutically.

22. a. What is cyclic AMP and what is its intracellular role in signal-transduction?

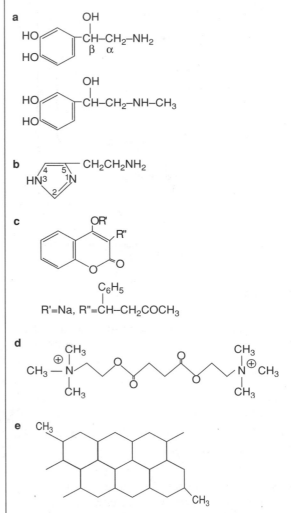

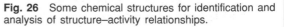

Fig. 26 Some chemical structures for identification and analysis of structure–activity relationships.

Describe and compare the roles of cyclic AMP in:

(i) noradrenaline action on the heart

(ii) the release of noradrenaline from the noradrenergic neuron

(iii) the effect of acetylcholine on the heart

(iv) the action of adrenaline on bronchial smooth muscle

(v) the action of theophylline on bronchial muscle.

b. List the hormones/drugs which increase or decrease cAMP.

23. A patient has recovered from an episode of myocardial infarction due to coronary thrombosis, and is now so terrified that he may have another attack that he has totally altered his lifestyle, reducing himself to zombie-like passivity. What pharmacological agent could be of value?

24. Indicate whether the statement below is true or false for the agents listed.

'The drugs given below have proved to be useful antimigraine drugs' (if the answer is true, name the drugs):

A. A 5-HT$_1$ agonist

B. A 5-HT$_2$ antagonist

C. A 5-HT$_1$ partial agonist

D. A 5-HT$_3$ antagonist

E. A 5-HT$_2$ partial agonist

F. A cyclo-oxygenase inhibitor.

25. What drugs could be useful in preventing migraine?

26. Are there good reasons for any of the following statements, and if so, what are they?

A. Patients with rheumatoid arthritis, who are being treated with penicillamine, should not, if they develop dyspepsia, take antacids at the same time as their penicillamine tablets.

B. Diabetic patients on chlorpropamide should be warned about the possible adverse effects of alcoholic drinks.

C. Anaemic patients taking ferrous gluconate should not take strong tea to help them swallow their iron tablets.

D. Patients on tetracyclines should not take their tablets after a milky drink.

E. Patients on MAO-inhibitors should avoid pickled herring.

F. Patients on penicillin should not eat Brussels sprouts.

27. A patient with severe rheumatoid joint disease needs to take regular doses of NSAIDs to alleviate pain and stiffness. Would problems of prescribing adequate therapy arise if such a patient were to develop one of the conditions listed below, and if so, what might be a pharmacological solution to the problem?

a. peptic ulcer

b. renal disease with impairment of function.

28. **a.** What is the anatomical and physiological basis for the analgesia produced by opiates as compared to that produced by NSAIDs?

b. What targets/receptors are affected by (i) opiates; (ii) NSAIDs?

29. From a report in the British Medical Journal: 'Five people ate the leaves of a South American plant which is grown as an ornamental shrub in Europe. They became ill shortly afterwards, the symptoms and signs being as follows: dilated pupils, anxiety, disorientation, visual hallucinations and delirium, dryness of the mouth, tachycardia, fever.'

On the basis of your knowledge of pharmacology work out:

What the active principle(s) in the leaves could have been?

What could have been the mechanism of action?

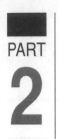

PART

2

What drug could be used as an antidote and how would it work?

Would you use a phenothiazine to decrease the CNS effects?

30. Give examples of four drugs whose clinical action involves a direct effect on ion channels. Specify which ion channels are affected and what the effects of drug action are. Outline the main clinical use(s) of the drugs you mention.

31. An individual is found unconscious after having injected an unknown drug intravenously. His breathing is slow, stertorous and wheezing; his blood pressure is low; his pupils are very small and he has regurgitated his gastric contents. What facts about this description give a clue as to what the drug might have been? Would a chemical examination of the gastric contents help in finding out what the drug was? What antidote might be effective in overcoming the CNS depression?

32. Using the simple diagram of the noradrenergic neuron in Figures 7 and 8 [see pp. 26, 29], give examples of the drugs in each of the groups which modify events at the sites indicated, taking the target cell as a smooth muscle cell. Outline the main clinical uses (if any) of each drug specified. (Note that the target cell is smooth muscle, not heart or CNS.)

33. Indicate whether the following interactions occur, and if so, how. Specify any deleterious or clinically useful consequences.

A. Aspirin increases the effect of warfarin.

B. Tranylcypromine decreases the effect of amphetamine.

C. Aspirin increases the effect of tolbutamide.

D. Terbutaline increases the effect of endogenous LTD_4 on bronchial muscle.

E. Tricyclic antidepressants and monoamine oxidase inhibitors given together may cause deleterious effects.

34. Give the main actions of the following compounds and state whether their clinically desirable effects are increased by metabolism to an active metabolite: prednisone, lithium, azathioprine, methicillin, cyclophosphamide, glyceryl trinitrate, paracetamol.

35. **a.** Describe or express diagrammatically:

the action of autonomic transmitters at the junction between autonomic nerves and cardiac tissues;

the receptors and transduction mechanisms involved;

drugs which could influence the processes which occur.

Specify which is the most important group of drugs, and what they are used for.

b. Some agents, whose actions elsewhere might be thought to be of value in treating hypertension, are not in fact useful for this purpose because of their effect in this region. Which agents are these and what action makes them unsuitable for general antihypertensive therapy?

36. Figure 27 shows, schematically, two notional neuronal terminals of:

- a projection neuron releasing the excitatory transmitter, glutamate, which is acting on a postsynaptic neuron, and causing excitation, and

- an inhibitory interneuron, releasing the inhibitory transmitter, GABA, which is acting on a postsynaptic neuron causing inhibition.

Also shown is a glial cell.

What is the precursor of GABA? What happens to GABA after it has been released? What receptors do GABA and glutamate act on and what are the main transduction mechanisms triggered by receptor activation? What drugs could influence the events occurring at the receptors and what might the drugs be used for clinically?

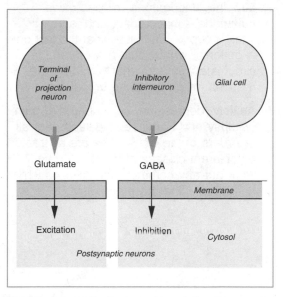

Fig. 27 Schematic diagram of two notional neuronal terminals in the CNS showing a projection neuron, releasing an excitatory transmitter, e.g. glutamate, and an inhibitory interneuron, releasing the inhibitory transmitter GABA. Also shown is a glial cell.

37. Which eicosanoid(s) are important in normal vascular endothelium/platelet interactions? Outline briefly the role of eicosanoids in the specific interaction between platelets and atherosclerotic plaque. Specify the likely result of the interaction in, e.g. the coronary circulation. How might drugs modify the processes you describe?

38. Some drugs are used to combat the side effects or the toxic effects of other drugs. State which drug(s) in Group A (if any) are used in the treatment of the unwanted effects of the agent(s) in Group B.

A. Pralidoxime, protamine sulphate, tranexamic acid, nalorphine, carbidopa, atropine, mesna, naloxone, methionine, vitamin K$_1$, neostigmine, desferrioxamine.

B. Morphine, dyflos, warfarin, suxamethonium, heparin, ferrous sulphate, streptokinase, paracetamol, levodopa, cyclophosphamide, tubocurarine.

39. Indicate whether the following statements are true or false. If you think a statement is false, explain why. In the presence of impaired renal function, the following statements would apply:

A. The dosage of many penicillin preparations would need to be reduced.

B. The effect of atenolol would, for practical purposes, be unchanged.

C. The effect of labetalol would, for practical purposes, be unchanged.

D. It would not be necessary to reduce the dosage of cephalosporins.

E. Cromoglycate would have a markedly enhanced effect.

F. Aminoglycosides would have toxic effects.

G. Ethanol, taken socially, would cumulate and there would be a marked increase in its plasma concentration.

40. Give examples of drugs that act by inhibiting the phosphodiesterase which metabolises cAMP, and outline the various conditions for which they might be useful.

41. Indicate which of the following statements are false and which true. If you think a statement is false, explain why.

A. 5-HT is a transmitter in the CNS.

B. An unwanted effect of codeine is diarrhoea.

C. The H$_1$-receptor antagonists, terfenadine and astemizole, have sedative actions.

D. The CNS stimulant, dexamphetamine, can improve intellectual performance in examinations if taken in substantial dosage.

E. Glycine is an inhibitory transmitter in the spinal cord.

F. Phenobarbitone is used as an intravenous anaesthetic.

G. The antiepileptic drug, carbamaze-pine, is used to treat absence seizures.

H. The muscarinic receptor antagonist, hyoscine, can be used to prevent motion sickness because it crosses the blood–brain barrier and prevents acetylcholine action on muscarinic receptors in the vomiting centre and related structures.

I. A combination of paracetamol with dextropropoxyphene is a safe analgesic for an over-the-counter preparation, combining as it does the advantage of a safe and effective NSAID with a safe and potent narcotic analgesic.

J. The effect of prolonged treatment with haloperidol is a decrease in activity of dopaminergic neurons and a proliferation of dopamine receptors associated with supersensitivity to dopamine.

K. Ethanol:

(i) is metabolised by first-order kinetics.

(ii) is distributed throughout the extracellular fluid.

(iii) impairs hand–eye coordination at levels above 80 mg/100 ml.

(iv) makes subjects constipated—they cannot pass pubs.

(v) improves intellectual performance.

42. What would be the consequences of antagonising:

a. fast excitatory transmission in the CNS

b. fast inhibitory transmission?

Give an example of the transmitters and receptors involved and a drug which is an antagonist in each case.

43. Could the glutamate and GABA systems in the CNS be useful targets for new, clinically useful drugs?

44. A patient was given the following sequence of drugs: diazepam, morphine, atropine, thiopentone, nitrous oxide, halothane, tubocurarine, and, some time later, a cup of tea. Given that the last one is optional, what would have been the circumstances and what would be the reasons for giving these drugs?

45. Anxiety, depression, schizophrenia, pain, epilepsy and Parkinson's disease are all disorders of the CNS. They are all treated by different classes of drugs. Can you work out any common principles which might underline the therapies?

Answers

1. Frusemide is a potassium-losing diuretic, and decreased plasma potassium increases digitalis toxicity. Addition of a potassium-sparing diuretic is necessary [see 🗐 pp. 374, 284, 378 box].

2. Glucocorticoids are synthesised and released as required and the process is very rapid. ACTH or tetracosactrin can cause synthesis and release within minutes [see 🗐 Fig. 21.13].

   The thyroid gland stores a 2–3 weeks' supply of the thyroid hormones. Consequently the response to drugs which inhibit their synthesis and are used to treat hyperthyroidism (e.g. carbimazole and other thioureylenes) may take weeks or months to produce an effect [see 🗐 Fig. 21.12]. (Iodine in large doses can decrease symptoms in 1–2 days and may be used temporarily in thyrotoxic crises.)

3. The effects would be due to the anticholinesterase action of the highly lipid-soluble organophosphate. This would bind covalently to the esteratic site of the enzyme, and so would cause excess acetylcholine action at both nicotinic and muscarinic receptors, respiratory effects being seen first in this case [see 🗐 p. 144 box].

   Peripheral muscarinic effects: bronchospasm and increased nasal, salivary and bronchial secretions; tonic constriction of the pupil and of the ciliary muscle with pain in the eye due to the spasm. If absorbed—colic and diarrhoea; sweating; urination; bradycardia and hypotension [see 🗐 p. 128 box].

   Peripheral nicotinic effects: fasciculations, weakness and finally

paralysis of skeletal muscles [see 🗐 pp. 142–144].

CNS effects: vomiting, disorientation, convulsions, coma. Death due to the paralysis of respiration (combined peripheral and central effects) [see 🗐 pp. 142–144].

4. Aspirin will increase the actions of warfarin, sulphonylureas, antiepileptics and methotrexate and may increase the half-life of penicillin, indomethacin and chlorpropamide [see 🗐 p. 792, Table 42.4]. It reduces the effect of probenecid, sulphinpyrazone and spironolactone. The mechanisms involved are as follows:

   Aspirin's *antiplatelet* action will increase the possibility of bleeding with the anticoagulant, warfarin [see 🗐 p. 338]. Gastric bleeding in particular may occur because the decreased generation of cytoprotective PGE_2, will result in increased acid and decreased mucus secretion [see Fig. 35 and 🗐 pp. 251, 387 box, 389, Fig 19.2].

   Aspirin is 50% *bound to plasma protein.* If the dose is large enough, this can result in 50% of the binding sites being occupied [see 🗐 Table 4.1]. This will affect drugs such as tolbutamide, warfarin, methotrexate and some sulphonamides, which work at the plasma concentrations at which the binding to protein is approaching saturation [see 🗐 Fig. 4.5]. The free concentrations of these drugs will be increased and their action augmented. In the case of the sulphonylurea agent, tolbutamide, this means that its hypoglycaemic action could be augmented. The risk of bleeding with warfarin and of toxicity with the anticancer agent, methotrexate, may be increased [see 🗐 p. 792].

   Aspirin *inhibits the metabolism* of valproate and phenytoin and thus increases their antiepileptic effects.

   Aspirin *reduces* urate *excretion* and can interfere with the action of the uricosuric

155

drugs, probenecid and sulphinpyrazone. *It will exacerbate gout in its own right as* well as reducing the effectiveness of treatment with the above agents [see 🖉 p. 254].

The active metabolite of spironolactone, canrenone, is secreted into the renal tubule and competitively antagonises the action of aldosterone on the sodium channels in the luminal membrane. Aspirin *interferes with the renal secretion* of canrenone into the proximal tubule and thus reduces the effective concentration of this agent in the filtrate.

Patients taking any of the above drugs should be warned against casual purchase and ingestion of large doses of aspirin preparations.

5. **A.** The decrease in warfarin action by phenobarbitone is (**b**), pharmacokinetic antagonism [see 🖉 Table 42.2, p. 339].

   B. Dimercaprol action in poisoning by inorganic mercurial compounds is (**a**), chemical antagonism [see 🖉 p. 16].

   C. The action of nifedipine (a Ca^{2+} channel blocker) on NA-mediated vasoconstriction is (**d**), block of receptor–effector linkage [see 🖉 Fig. 14.1, pp. 302 box, 297 box].

   D. The effects of salbutamol (a β_2-agonist) on histamine-induced bronchoconstriction is (**e**), physiological antagonism [see 🖉 p. 360 box, Fig. 17.3].

   E. Phenoxybenzamine effect on NA-induced vasoconstriction is (**c** ii), irreversible (non-equilibrium) competitive receptor antagonism [see 🖉 Table 7.4].

   F. Trimetaphan on ACh-mediated stimulation in autonomic ganglia is (**d**), block of receptor–effector linkage [see 🖉 Fig. 6.6, pp. 17, 130].

   G. The action of cimetidine on histamine-induced gastric secretion is (**c** i), reversible, competitive receptor antagonism [see 🖉 Fig. 19.3A].

6. *Please don't, with your patient's complicity,*
   Write prescriptions with frank eccentricity.
   Steroid drugs in excess
   Given long term, no less,
   Would result in gross iatrogenicity.

   We hope you would refuse the patient's request, and insist not only on keeping the maintenance dose as low as possible but on careful monitoring of her condition. In other words, the drug therapy you should consider should be that already being given. Chronic administration of glucocorticoids can result in many adverse effects—susceptibility to infection, adrenal suppression, Cushing's-type syndrome [see 🖉 Fig. 21.16]. Sudden cessation of the drug could lead to acute adrenal insufficiency; this would be serious.

7. There may be an increased risk of bleeding from the peptic ulcer because: cimetidine potentiates the anticoagulant action of warfarin by inhibiting its metabolism [see 🖉 p. 338]; aspirin inhibits platelet activation mechanisms, reducing platelet aggregation by inhibiting cyclo-oxygenase and thus TXA_2 generation [see 🖉 Fig. 11.8, p. 344 box]; it also reduces PGE_2 formation in the gastric mucosa, removing the 'cytoprotective' effect of PGE_2. PGE_2 normally inhibits gastric acid secretion and stimulates mucus and bicarbonate secretion [see 🖉 Fig. 19.2, pp. 389, 393]. But note that death from pulmonary embolism in a patient with deep vein thrombosis is such an appreciable risk that heparin and warfarin would probably need to be used as the lesser of two unfortunate risks.

8. One species of LDL, lipoprotein(a), which is strongly associated with atherosclerosis and is localised in atheromatous plaques, carries a special apoprotein, apo(a). Apo(a) is very similar in structure to plasminogen; it competes with and inhibits the binding of plasminogen and thus reduces fibrinolysis [see 🖉 p. 324].

9. See Figure 28.

   a. Acetylcholine acts on nicotinic receptors in autonomic ganglia and on muscarinic M_3- and M_2-receptors in target organs and at postganglionic sites. M_1-receptors, found on the postsynaptic membranes in autonomic ganglia, may also be activated to produce slow

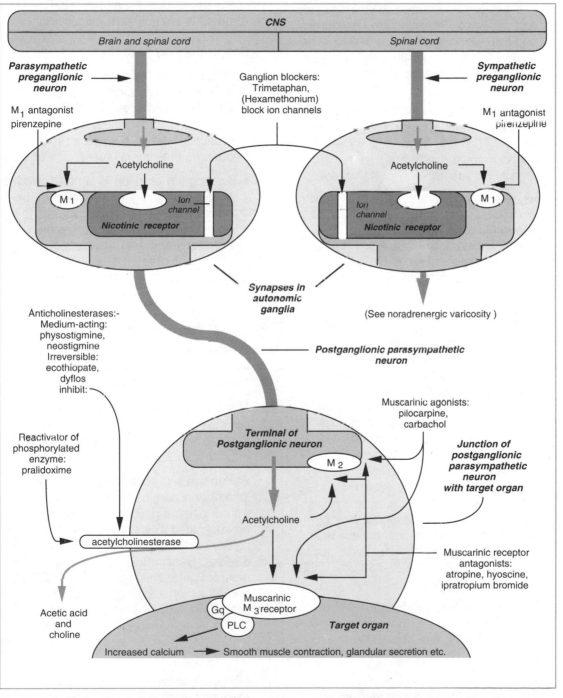

Fig. 28 Drugs affecting events at autonomic ganglia and the junction of postganglionic parasympathetic neuron with target organ. M_1, M_2, M_3 = muscarinic receptors; Gq = PLC-activating G-protein; PLC = phospholipase C.

excitation; they are selectively blocked by pirenzepine [see ✑ Table 6.1]. M_2-receptors are also found in cardiac tissue [see Fig. 33 and ✑ p. 120 box, Table 6.1].

Note that carbachol acts on nicotinic as well as muscarinic receptors (not shown). The sympathetic nerves to sweat glands and piloerector muscles are cholinergic and the events specified for the junction of postganglionic parasympathetic fibre and target organ will occur at these sites [see ✑ Fig. 5.5].

b. There are three main subclasses of muscarinic receptors [see ✑ p. 120 box, Table 6.1]. Drugs used clinically which act on, or give rise to action on muscarinic receptors are given below:

GIT: Bethanechol and carbachol, which are muscarinic agonists at M_3-receptors, and neostigmine, which is an anticholinesterase with medium duration of action, have been used in the treatment of postoperative GIT atony, but are now less frequently employed. Atropine, hyoscine, propantheline, non-selective M-receptor antagonists, given orally, are sometimes used for GIT disorders that have a component of spasm. Pirenzepine, an M_1-receptor antagonist, inhibits acetylcholine stimulation of postsynaptic M_1-receptors in parasympathetic ganglia and possibly also M_1-receptors on gastric parietal cells; it interferes with gastric acid secretion and is used, orally, in the treatment of peptic ulcer [see ✑ Ch. 19]. Dicyclomine, an M_1-receptor antagonist, which may have an additional direct relaxant action on smooth muscle is given orally for GIT disorders with spasm [see ✑ pp. 127, 128–129, 128 box, Table 6.1, Fig. 19.2, p. 392 box].

The urinary tract: Bethanechol and carbachol, which are muscarinic agonists at M_3-receptors, can be used in the treatment of postoperative urinary retention.

The eye: Pilocarpine and carbachol (muscarinic agonists at M_3-receptors),

physostigmine (medium-duration anticholinesterase) are used topically in the treatment of glaucoma. Homatropine, cyclopentolate and tropicamide are non-selective M_3-receptor antagonists used topically during ophthalmic examination of the retina [see ✑ pp. 126–127]. Atropine is also used in iridocyclitis.

Respiratory system:

- Atropine and hyoscine, non-selective M-receptor antagonists, are given parenterally in pre-anaesthetic medication to decrease reflex bronchial and salivary secretion during anaesthesia [see ✑ p. 128 box].

- Ipratropium bromide is a non-selective M-receptor antagonist which may be given by inhalation as an adjunct to β_2-adrenoceptor agonists in treatment of bronchitis and also the immediate phase of asthma if there is a component of parasympathetic-mediated bronchospasm (as in asthma triggered by irritant stimuli) [see ✑ p. 360 box].

Cardiovascular system: There are few clinical indications for the CVS effects of muscarinic agonists or antagonists.

Motion sickness: Hyoscine, a non-selective M-receptor antagonist, is given orally to prevent motion sickness [see ✑ Fig. 19.8, p. 395 box].

Parkinson's disease: Hyperactivity of striatal cholinergic neurons, associated with dopamine deficiency, is believed to be implicated in the symptom-complex of rigidity and hypokinesia of Parkinson's disease. Benztropine, a non-selective M-receptor antagonist (given orally or i.m.) and trihexyphenidyl, an M_1-receptor antagonist, are second-line drugs for treatment of parkinsonism (levodopa is first choice) [see ✑ pp. 129, 505 box, 530 box, 129].

10. Figure 29 shows a diagrammatic representation of the nephron in which the following are summarised:

(i) the areas where there are moderate or high salt concentrations in the interstitia [see 📖 Fig. 18.6];

(ii) the sites of action of the main diuretics (with their mechanisms of action indicated schematically) and a list of their

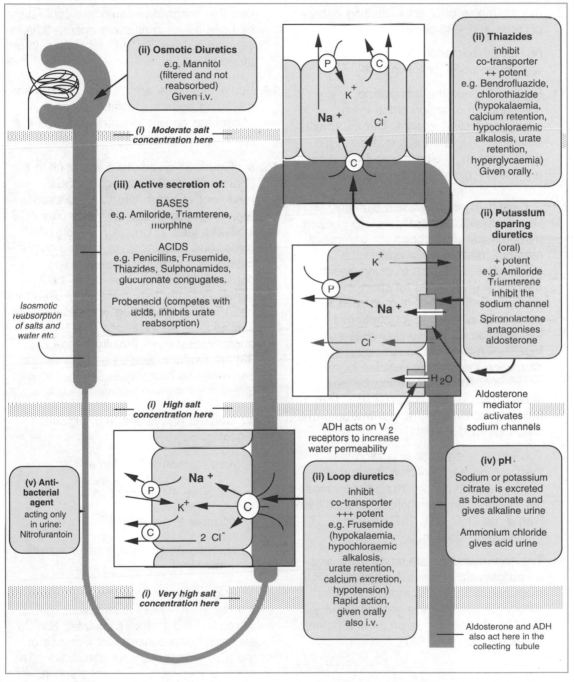

Fig. 29 Summary chart of drug action in the nephron, showing (i) areas of moderate, high and very high salt concentration; (ii) the principal diuretics; (iii) some of the main agents secreted into the proximal tubule; (iv) examples of drugs affecting pH; and (v) an antibacterial agent which acts specifically in the urine. C = co-transporter; P = sodium pump; ADH = antidiuretic hormone.

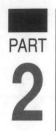

principal characteristics [see ✎ Figs 18.11, 18.13, 18.14];

(iii) the site of active secretion of drugs into the tubule, with some examples of agents secreted [see ✎ Table 4.5];

(iv) examples of agents affecting urinary pH [see ✎ p. 383 box];

(v) an antibacterial agent which acts only in the urine [see ✎ p. 738].

11. Figure 30 gives the names and mechanisms of action of the main antihypertensive* agents. The four most important drug groups are listed in the figure caption. β-blockers and diuretics are usually given together. ACE inhibitors are now often used as first-line therapy, but are best not given with diuretics. Drugs given parenterally include sodium nitroprusside (first choice for parenteral therapy), diazoxide, labetalol, hydralazine. Ganglion blocking agents (not shown) are used for short-term emergency treatment (e.g. for dissecting aortic aneurysm) and for controlled hypotension during surgery. Reserpine (not shown) decreases NA release by damaging the storage vesicles in the noradrenergic neuron varicosity [see ✎ Table 14.5, pp. 162 box, 164 box, 166 box, 174 box, Table 7.4, pp. 312 box, 378 box, Figs 18.13, 18.11].

12. You would need to bear in mind that theophylline has a narrow therapeutic window and that ciprofloxacin increases the plasma concentrations of theophylline [see ✎ pp. 360, 361, 757] whereas trimethoprim does not.

13. The common uses are as antacids and as purgatives. Magnesium hydroxide, magnesium trisilicate and magnesium carbonate are effective antacids [see ✎ p. 391]. Magnesium sulphate is a potent purgative [see ✎ p. 397]. Recent

evidence suggests that magnesium salts, i.v, may reduce mortality in patients with acute myocardial infarction (Br Med J Dec 1991, p. 303). A student (subsequently marked down for a flippant approach to therapeutics) suggested in a viva that magnesium sulphate could also be used as an antitussive agent—'after a very large dose, Sir, the patient would be afraid to cough'.

14. Some examples are: phenoxybenzamine; alkylating agents; cisplatin; organo-phosphate anticholinesterases ... [see ✎ pp. 163, 706 box, 141].

15. **a.** Figure 31 gives the drugs used in the pharmacological approach to the treatment of heart failure. A standard regime is digoxin plus diuretics plus ACE inhibitors [see ✎ Ch. 14]. The digitalis glycosides may increase cardiac output mainly by improving diastolic filling consequent on their slowing of the ventricular rate; they are mainly used for heart failure associated with atrial fibrillation. β-agonists and phosphodiesterase inhibitors [see Fig. 33] are useful in acute heart failure but can increase mortality in severe chronic failure.*

b. Cardiac glycosides, e.g. digoxin, digitoxin:

- increase contractile force

- decrease AV conduction

- increase vagal activity

- increase ectopic pacemaker activity (unwanted).

Their mechanism of action is inhibition of the Na^+/K^+-ATPase which results in increased $[Na^+]_i$. This stimulates Na^+/Ca^{2+} exchange and consequent increase of the $[Ca^{2+}]_i$ necessary for contraction. The effect is increased by hypokalaemia.

---

* You might find it enlightening to read an article in British Medical Journal of Feb 18, 1989, written by an electrical engineer, giving his personal experiences of the actions and side effects of antihypertensive drugs over a 39-year period.

* See N Engl J Med 325: 1505, 1991; Annu Rev Med 41: 65, 1990.

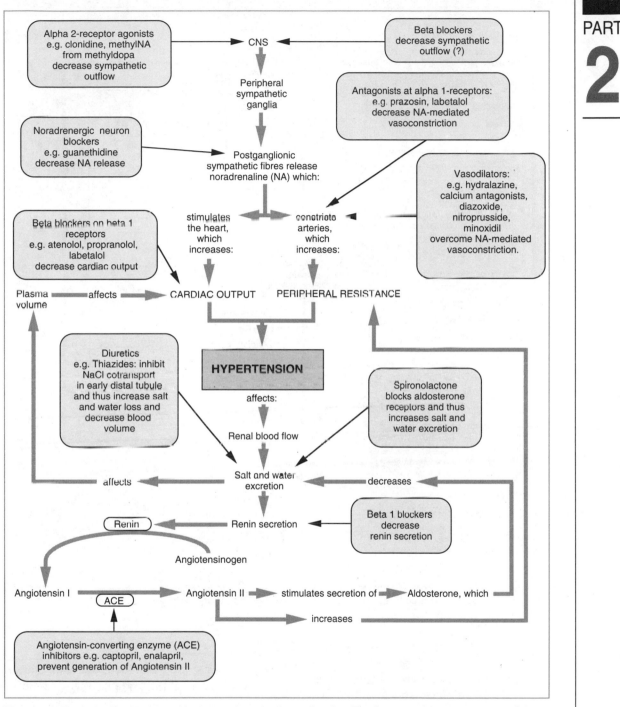

Fig. 30 Antihypertensive agents, with sites and mechanisms of action. The four most important groups of drugs are beta 1 blockers, diuretics, ACE inhibitors and vasodilators.

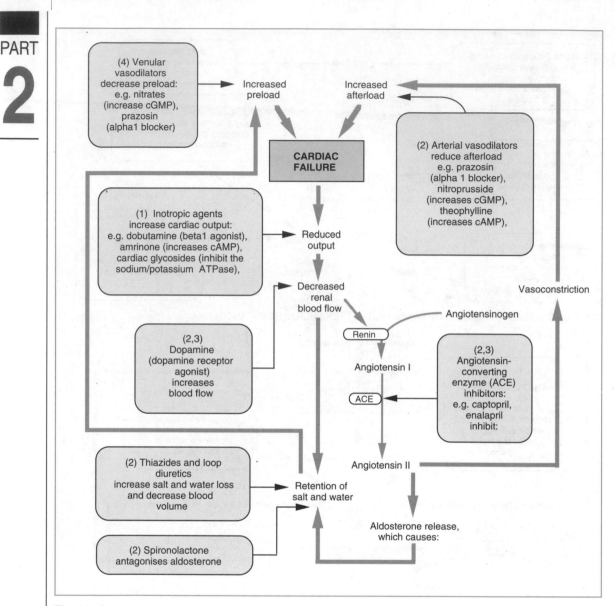

Fig. 31 Drugs used in the treatment of heart failure. The aims of therapy are: (a) to increase contractility and thus cardiac output (Group 1 drugs do this); (b) to reduce afterload (Groups 2 and 3 do this); (c) to decrease preload (Groups 3 and 4 do this).

Unwanted actions: dysrhythmias, nausea, anorexia, visual disturbances, potential heart block [see ▱ p. 285 box].

ACE inhibitors, given orally, reduce blood pressure and cardiac afterload and decrease aldosterone secretion, which results in less Na⁺ retention, decreased plasma volume and hence decreased preload [see ▱ p. 315].

Thiazides, loop diuretics, spironolactone: see Figure 29 [also ▱ pp. 377, 379–380].

Dobutamine, in moderate doses, is inotropic by action on β_1-receptors in the heart [see Fig. 33 and ▱ p. 285]. In addition, it acts on dopamine receptors in renal, mesenteric and coronary blood vessels to cause vasodilatation; the effect on renal blood vessels resulting in an increase in glomerular filtration rate and increased natriuresis. (Higher doses stimulate α_1-receptors and cause vasoconstriction) [see Ch. 41 and 📖 p. 309].

Prazosin: see Figure 32.

16. The drug could be either a muscarinic receptor agonist or histamine, but could not be any of the others.

A muscarinic receptor agonist such as acetylcholine or carbachol would:

- reduce blood pressure by stimulating M_3-receptors on vascular endothelium producing relaxation (mainly by direct action but partly by releasing nitric oxide) and also by stimulating M_2-receptors in the heart, reducing cardiac output [see 📖 Table 7.1, Fig. 14.1].

- contract guinea-pig ileum and constrict bronchi by stimulating M_3-receptors on smooth muscle thus increasing intracellular calcium [see 📖 Table 6.1, pp. 355 box, 128 box].

Histamine would reduce blood pressure by a combined effect on H_1- and H_2-receptors; H_2-receptors activate adenylate cyclase causing relaxation of vascular muscle and it is possible that the H_1-mediated vasodilatation is due to the release of EDRF. It would contract ileum and constrict bronchi by stimulating H_1-receptors on smooth muscle thus increasing intracellular calcium [see 📖 pp. 227, 229 box].

Adrenaline would increase blood pressure by an action on vascular α_1-receptors if the pressure was normal or low, but could reduce it by an action on vascular β_2-receptors if the pressure was high. It would not cause contraction of ileum or constriction of bronchi [see 📖 p. 151 box, 355 box, Table 5.1].

An α_1-adrenoceptor antagonist might reduce blood pressure but would not contract the isolated guinea-pig ileum. It would not cause bronchoconstriction [see 📖 Fig. 17.1].

A β-adrenoceptor antagonist might reduce blood pressure by reducing cardiac output but would not contract guinea-pig ileum. Given on its own, it usually has no effect on bronchi [see 📖 pp. 164 box, 166 box, Fig. 17.1]. But note that in an asthmatic patient, endogenous circulating adrenaline would be opposing the action of spasmogenic mediators by acting as a physiological antagonist; in this situation, a β-receptor antagonist would prevent the relaxant action of endogenous adrenaline, resulting in bronchoconstriction by the now unopposed spasmogens.

It would be possible to determine whether X was histamine or a muscarinic agonist by testing the effect of specific antagonists on the smooth muscle action of X. An H_1-receptor blocker, such as mepyramine, should competitively antagonise histamine, and atropine should competitively antagonise a muscarinic agonist.

More information could be obtained if it were possible to apply the drug to the eye; a muscarinic agonist would cause pupillary constriction.

17. Sulphonamides interfere with the synthesis of folate, and folate antagonists interfere with the utilisation of folate. These agents are made use of in the chemotherapy of bacterial infection and malaria, the antibacterial folate antagonist being trimethoprim and the antimalarial, pyrimethamine. The folate antagonist, methotrexate, is used in cancer treatment. Folate itself is used to treat megaloblastic anaemia, if this is due to folate deficiency [see 📖 pp. 683–684, Table 35.1, p. 721, Fig. 37.2, p. 708 box, Figs 36.7, 36.8, p. 483 box].

18. a. The drugs most commonly used to treat hypertension are β_1-blockers, diuretics and vasodilators [see Fig. 30]. The diuretics most commonly used in hypertension are thiazides, though loop diuretics may also be used. Both these groups of diuretics cause a decrease in

uric acid excretion and can precipitate gout; and the clinical signs and symptoms presented by the patient are typical of gout.

b. Drugs used to treat gout: for short-term treatment of the acute attack and to alleviate the pain, an NSAID is used. Indomethacin would be the drug of choice; salicylates would exacerbate the condition because they decrease uric acid excretion [see 📖 p. 254]. For long-term treatment, drugs which inhibit uric acid synthesis (allopurinol) or uricosuric agents (probenecid, sulphinpyrazone) may be used, but treatment is postponed for several weeks as these drugs can trigger further episodes of gout. Probably the best anti-gout drug in this patient would be colchicine [see 📖 pp. 258, 259].

19. Analysis of structure–activity relationships is of value for the understanding of how drugs work, is crucial for the rational development of new drugs and can contribute to solving problems of receptor classification. The more esoteric chemical aspects of the study of structure–activity are the province of the medicinal chemist and are beyond the scope of this book. However, even a fairly superficial study of the chemical formulae of some compounds can be informative and can enhance understanding of basic pharmacology. But our view is that it is rather a waste of time for medical students and most pharmacology students to memorise structures (e.g. erythromycin) which do nothing towards this end.

a. The structures are noradrenaline and adrenaline. It is of value to know this because the knowledge facilitates understanding of the relationships between noradrenergic transmitters and drugs which mimic or modify their actions. Analysis of the effects of adrenaline, noradrenaline, and a synthetic catecholamine, isoprenaline (in particular the rank order of the potencies

of these agents for different activities) led to the understanding that there were several types of adrenoceptor. When modified in different ways, these molecules yield compounds that have different actions on adrenoceptors and/or on the noradrenergic neuron varicosity, e.g. the indirectly acting sympathomimetic amines, selective α-agonists, selective β-agonists, selective β-antagonists [see 📖 Fig. 7.7].

b. The structure is histamine. Analysis of the actions of histamine and the effects of early antihistamine drugs led Ash and Schild to propose that there were two types of histamine receptor in the body; they labelled the antihistamine used (mepyramine) an 'H$_1$-receptor antagonist'. Subsequent work by Black and his colleagues with modified versions of the histamine molecule resulted in the development of H$_2$-receptor agonists and antagonists. Drugs acting on putative H$_3$-receptors have now been described [see 📖 Tables 11.1a, 11.1b, 12.4].

c. The structure is warfarin. There is a structural similarity between warfarin and vitamin K and its congeners. This similarity is the basis for the inhibitory action of warfarin on the enzymes which normally reduce vitamin K and make it available as a cofactor for other enzymes which carboxylate glutamic acid residues in factors II, VII, IX and X, thus conferring on them the Ca^{2+}-binding properties essential for their interaction in the coagulation cascade [see 📖 Figs 16.3–16.5].

d. The structure is suxamethonium, a depolarising neuromuscular blocking drug [see 📖 Table 6.4]. It consists essentially of two acetylcholine molecules linked by their acetyl groups [see 📖 Table 6.2]. It is sufficiently similar to acetylcholine for it to act on the endplate of skeletal muscle just like acetylcholine; but it acts for long enough to cause loss of electrical excitability (due to the voltage-sensitive sodium channels becoming inactivated and no longer able to open in response to the depolarising stimulus). The structural relationship to acetylcholine is sufficiently close for suxamethonium to be a substrate for plasma cholinesterase. It is hydrolysed rapidly by this enzyme and consequently has a very short duration of action, of about 3 minutes [see 🖊 p. 139 box].

e. This compound is 'dimethylchicken wire'.

20. Acetylcholine causes contraction of both, acting on nicotinic receptors in skeletal muscle, but on muscarinic M_3-receptors in GIT smooth muscle. The nicotinic receptor is a ligand-gated ion channel. The M_3-receptor is a G-protein-coupled receptor causing activation of phospholipase C, an enzyme that acts on PIP_2 to give rise to $InsP_3$ (which mobilises Ca^{2+}) and DAG (which activates PKC) [see 🖊 p. 120 box, Table 6.1].

21. **a.** Competitive antagonists are known for angiotensin II, bombesin, bradykinin, cholecystokinin, GnRH, opioid peptides, oxytocin, substance P, vasoactive intestinal peptide and vasopressin [see 🖊 Table 9.1].

b. Naloxone is an opioid receptor antagonist used for morphine overdose. Vasopressin (ADH) is used to treat diabetes insipidus. Oxytocin is used to induce labour and to treat postpartum haemorrhage. Saralasin is a competitive inhibitor of the vasoconstrictor action of angiotensin II and may be of value in treating hypertension. (Note that its inhibitory effect is due to the fact that it is a partial agonist rather than a true competitive antagonist) [see 🖊 pp. 631, 424 box, 472 box, 316].

22. **a.** Cyclic AMP (cAMP) is a nucleotide, derived from ATP by the action of adenylate cyclase. It is a messenger operated by G-protein-coupled receptors. In many cells, two G-proteins, with opposite functions, can interact with adenylate cyclase: G_s stimulates the enzymes thus increasing cAMP, G_i

inhibits it thus decreasing cAMP. The concentration of cAMP is determined not only by the effects of these G-proteins, but also by the action of a phosphodiesterase which converts cAMP into AMP. cAMP activates a kinase—termed the cyclic AMP-dependent kinase or protein kinase A (PKA)—which phosphorylates other intracellular proteins (enzymes, ion channels), thereby regulating their function [see 🖊 p. 36].

(i) Noradrenaline acts on β_1-receptors in the heart to cause increased rate, increased force of contraction and facilitation of AV conduction, the action being mainly if not entirely due to an increase in cAMP brought about by G_s activation of adenylate cyclase. Cyclic AMP activates PKA which phosphorylates membrane calcium channels. The result is an increase in the number of channels which open in response to a given depolarisation and thus an increase in the rise in internal calcium which accompanies the action potential [see 🖊 p. 280 box].

(ii) The release of noradrenaline from the noradrenergic neuron varicosity is triggered by the influx of calcium through the voltage-dependent calcium channels that open as a result of the depolarisation caused by the action potential. Stimulation of the presynaptic α_2-receptors inhibits calcium entry and noradrenaline release. There is some evidence that the opening of the calcium channels is brought about by increased cAMP as in the heart (see above), and that α_2-G_i-mediated inhibition of adenylate cyclase results in decreased cAMP and thus decreased calcium entry [see 🖊 Fig. 7.4]. However, there is another suggestion that α_2-receptors interact with G-proteins which directly control the calcium channels.

(iii) Acetylcholine causes slowing of the heart rate, decreased force of contraction and inhibition of AV conduction, by an action on muscarinic M_2-receptors. These receptors are negatively coupled to adenylate cyclase by inhibitory G_i-proteins which decrease adenylate cyclase activity and reduce the cAMP concentration, thus inhibiting calcium entry [cf. (i) above]. M_2-receptors are also coupled to G-proteins which directly open K^+ channels [see Fig. 33 and 📖 p. 282].

(iv) Adrenaline acts on β-receptors to relax bronchial muscle. $β_2$-receptors are coupled via a stimulatory G-protein to adenylate cyclase, which, when stimulated, increases the cAMP concentration. Cyclic AMP activates PKA which:

- phosphorylates myosin-light-chain kinase (MLCK), inactivating it and thus interfering with the MLCK-mediated phosphorylation of myosin essential for contraction

- promotes Ca^{2+} efflux by an action on the membrane Ca^{2+} pump, thus lowering $[Ca^{2+}]_i$. Intracellular Ca^{2+} is the main internal messenger for contraction [see Fig. 22].

Recent work has shown that PKA also:

- inhibits PIP_2 hydrolysis

- increases Ca^{2+} uptake into the sarcoplasmic reticulum

- activates K^+ channels, causing hyperpolarisation and reduced excitability.

(v) Theophylline relaxes bronchial muscle by inhibiting the phosphodiesterase which converts cAMP to AMP; it thus increases the concentration of cAMP with the consequences outlined in (iv) above [see Fig. 22 and 📖 p. 360].

b. Agents which increase cAMP include: $β_2$-adrenoceptor agonists, glucagon, antidiuretic hormone on renal tubule cells, gonadotrophins, corticotrophin, corticotrophin-releasing hormone, parathormone, thyrotrophin, adenosine, prostacyclin, PGE_2 on EP_2-receptors, PGD_2, dopamine (on renal and

mesenteric vasculature). All these increase cAMP by an action on G_s-coupled receptors; xanthines increase cAMP by inhibiting its metabolism to AMP [see above].

Agents which decrease cAMP include: muscarinic M_2-receptor agonists, $α_2$-adrenoceptor agonists, opioids on δ-receptors.

23. *If a heart attack patient supposes*
That he'll suffer another thrombosis
Quarter aspirin a day
Should keep infarcts at bay
And alleviate heart-linked neurosis.

[See 📖 p. 348 box].

24. **A.** True; sumatriptan [see 📖 p. 187 box].

B. True; methysergide, pizotifen, cyproheptadine. Pizotifen and cyproheptadine are useful in prevention, not treatment; they also have some H_1-antagonist actions. Methysergide can have serious unwanted effects (fibrosis of pleura, peritoneum, heart valves) and should only be given under hospital supervision [see 📖 pp. 187 box, 261].

C. True; methysergide [but see (ii) above and 📖 Table 8.1].

D. True; ondansetron [see 📖 Table 8.1].

E. True; ergotamine, which is also a partial agonist at $α_1$-adrenoceptors. It is useful in the treatment of migraine but note that it may increase vomiting since it can in its own right cause nausea and vomiting [see 📖 pp. 184, 187 box, Table 8.2].

F. True; aspirin, paracetamol [see 📖 p. 249].

(It would seem that 5-HT is involved in the pathogenesis of migraine.)

25. Pizotifen, β-blockers.

26. **A.** Yes; penicillamine is a metal chelator [see 📖 p. 257]; antacids reduce its absorption.

B. Yes; the combination could cause unpleasant nausea, headache and unseemly flushing [see 📖 p. 414].

C. Yes; the tannates in tea might inhibit iron absorption [see 📖 p. 477].

D. Yes; absorption of tetracyclines (which chelate metal ions) is decreased in the presence of milk [see 📖 p. 730].

E. Yes; pickled herring contains tyramine which releases NA from noradrenergic neurons. Normally released NA is taken back into the neuron by uptake 1 where some is metabolised in the cytosol by MAO bound to the surface of mitochondria and the rest is taken up into the vesicles [see Fig. 32]. MAO inhibitors prevent the metabolism of NA in the neuron, increasing the NA content of the vesicle and enhancing sympathomimetic effects. A further, and probably important action of MAO inhibitors is exerted in the GIT and the liver, in both of which there are high concentrations of MAO. Tyramine in food normally undergoes substantial deamination in GIT and liver so that very little enters the circulation. In the presence of MAO inhibitors, much greater amounts get into the circulation and eventually reach the noradrenergic neurons where they are taken up by uptake 1 [see 📖 Table 7.3]. Patients on MAO inhibitors who eat cheese, pickled herring, Marmite, Bovril and other tyramine-containing foods, run a risk of precipitating a hypertensive crisis due to the action of released NA on blood vessels and heart.

F. No; only the reasons put forward by the Vegetable Liberation Front (reputed to be based in Belgium).

27. a. NSAIDs are likely to exacerbate the gastric damage of peptic ulcer because they prevent the local synthesis of cytoprotective prostaglandins [see 📖 pp. 387 box, 252 box]. H_2-receptor antagonists (which might anyway be being used for treatment of the peptic ulcer) would reduce such acid secretion.

But an additional potential pharmacological solution would be to use misoprostol, an analogue of PGE_2 which acts on EP_3-receptors on mucosal cells inhibiting gastric acid secretion and promoting mucus and bicarbonate secretion [see Fig. 13].

b. Renal prostaglandins have a role in the local regulation of blood flow, glomerular filtration and the handling of salt and water [see 📖 p. 375]. NSAIDs, by decreasing PG production, are likely to exacerbate renal impairment. There is no really adequate pharmacological solution to this problem other than to reduce the dose of NSAID as far as possible while monitoring renal function.

28. The targets for opiates are μ-, δ- and κ-receptors [see 📖 Table 31.3] whereas the target for NSAIDs is the cyclo-oxygenase which acts on arachidonate to give rise to the prostanoids [see 📖 Figs 11.5, 11.8]. The primary afferent nociceptor is a bipolar neuron with cell body in the dorsal horn, peripheral axon in the periphery and central axon terminating in the dorsal horn of the spinal cord [see 📖 p. 613]. The peripheral axon (pain C fibre) is activated by noxious stimuli, the effect being caused and/or exacerbated by sensitisation by the mediators (Bk, PGs, LTs) generated by inflammation and tissue damage [see 📖 pp. 614–615, Fig. 31.5]. The primary nociceptive neuron relays both to the thalamus and cortex and to motor neurons via second-order nociceptive neurons. Opioid receptors are concentrated at two sites, on the terminal of the central axon of the primary nociceptive neurons and in the midbrain; and opiate action at these sites constitutes spinal and supraspinal analgesia respectively [see Fig. 18]. They are also present on neurons of the enteric nervous system and it is these which are responsible for the action of opiates on the GIT [see 📖 Table 31.2]. NSAIDs, by inhibiting PG production, decrease the sensitisation of the peripheral nerve endings of the

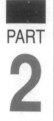

PART

2

nociceptive neurons [see Fig. 18 and 🖉 pp. 248–249].

29. The active principles were belladonna alkaloids, mainly atropine in this instance. The mechanism of action was by competitive antagonism of acetylcholine at muscarinic receptors [see 🖉 p. 128 box]. Note that hyoscine has CNS depressant actions. If an antidote were necessary (after gastric lavage) physostigmine would be given parenterally, i.e. the reversible anticholinesterase which is least ionised at body pH and will thus pass into the CNS [see 🖉 pp. 140, 144].

Phenothiazines have varying degrees of atropine-like activity and could make matters worse [see 🖉 Table 28.1]; a benzodiazepine could be used as a sedative.

30. You could have chosen from the following:

Local anaesthetics, e.g. lignocaine, which blocks voltage-gated Na⁺ channels in neurons, preventing action potential generation. It is given by injection or infiltration for local effect, injection for nerve block and spinal or epidural anaesthesia and topically for surface anaesthesia. Elimination is 95% by metabolism in the liver [see Fig. 19 and 🖉 Table 28.1].

Amiloride blocks the Na⁺ channels on the luminal membrane of the collecting tubule of the nephron, thus preventing the action of aldosterone's protein mediator which normally increases Na⁺ uptake from the filtrate. It is a potassium-sparing diuretic often used in conjunction with thiazides or loop diuretics to offset their potassium-losing effects. Another similar drug is triamterene [see Fig. 29 and 🖉 p. 378 box].

Diltiazem, a calcium antagonist, binds to the L-type voltage-gated Ca²⁺ channels on vascular smooth muscle and cardiac muscle, preventing channel opening. In cardiac muscle this results in AV block and thus cardiac slowing and decreased

contractility; in smooth muscle (particularly arteriolar smooth muscle) it results in vasodilatation. Diltiazem is used to treat angina, hypertension and cardiac dysrhythmias. Similar drugs are nifedipine (more active on blood vessels than heart), verapamil (more active on heart than blood vessels) [see Fig. 10 and 🖉 p. 297 box].

Benzodiazepines, e.g. diazepam, which binds to a specific regulatory site on the GABAₐ receptor on neurons in the CNS; it increases the affinity of the receptor for GABAₐ, resulting in an increase in the number of Cl⁻ channels which are opened by a given concentration of GABA. The increased influx of Cl⁻ causes hyperpolarisation of the membrane, and the result is neuronal inhibition. Diazepam is used as an anxiolytic and hypnotic, and also as an anticonvulsant (in status epilepticus and poison-induced convulsions), for various types of muscle spasm, for pre-anaesthetic medication and for sedation during minor operative procedures [see 🖉 Table 27.1 for other examples, pp. 552–553, Fig. 27.4].

Sulphonylureas, e.g. tolbutamide, which inhibits the ATP-sensitive K⁺ channels in the membrane of pancreatic β-cells. These K⁺ channels are important in regulating insulin release. When the cellular ATP concentration falls, the channels open causing hyperpolarisation and decreased insulin secretion. Blocking the channel causes the cells to depolarise leading to Ca²⁺ influx which stimulates insulin release. Tolbutamide is used to treat non-insulin-dependent diabetes [see 🖉 p. 415, Table 20.4 for other examples].

Minoxidil antagonises the action of ATP on ATP-sensitive K⁺ channels in vascular smooth muscle cells permitting K⁺ efflux and membrane hyperpolarisation; this results in vasodilatation. Minoxidil is used for severe hypertension. Other examples are cromakalim, pinacidil, diazoxide [see 🖉 pp. 310–311].

31. The patient's condition suggests that the drug was morphine or a morphine-like drug, since these agents in overdose cause serious CNS depression with respiratory depression and constricted pupils [see ✏ p. 624 box] but stimulate the chemoreceptor trigger zone in the medulla to cause vomiting [see ✏ p. 393]. Morphine causes histamine release which produces bronchoconstriction [see ✏ p. 624]; this could cause wheezing respiration. The morphine is very likely to be present in the gastric contents, since, being a weak base, it can undergo ion trapping in the stomach [see Fig. 5 and ✏ p. 69, Fig. 4.4]. An effective antidote would be naloxone [see ✏ p. 631 box].

32. Figure 32 gives examples of the drugs which affect the events at the junction of noradrenergic neuron and a smooth muscle cell. (If the figure strikes you as hideously complex, avert your eyes and pass on to Question 33.)

Clinical uses of the drugs in Figure 32 are as follows:

Agents acting on receptors:

α-agonist, adrenaline: vasoconstrictor with local anaesthetic injection; for anaphylactic shock [see ✏ p. 162 box].

α_1-agonist, dopamine: this acts mainly on dopamine receptors causing relaxation of mesenteric vessels but can cause contraction of other vascular muscle by acting on α_1-receptors; it is infused to raise blood pressure in hypovolaemic shock (also causes increased cardiac contraction by stimulating β_1-receptors) [see ✏ Ch. 14, p. 309].

α_1-agonist, phenylephrine: nasal decongestant [see ✏ Table 7.4].

α_1-agonist, methoxamine: to overcome hypotension during anaesthesia [see ✏ Table 7.4, p. 162 box].

α_1-antagonist, prazosin: for hypertension [see ✏ Table 14.5].

α_1-antagonist, ergotamine: for migraine [see ✏ Table 8.2].

α_1-antagonist, phenoxybenzamine: used with β-blocker for temporary treatment of the hypertension caused by phaeochromocytoma (the main treatment is surgical removal of the tumour) [see ✏ p. 164].

α_2-agonist, clonidine: for hypertension. (But its main locus of action is probably in the CNS) [see ✏ Tables 7.4, 14.4, p. 162 box].

β_2-agonists, salbutamol and terbutaline: by inhalation as bronchodilators in asthma; as uterine relaxants in premature labour [see ✏ pp. 359, 470].

β_2-agonist, adrenaline: for acute anaphylactic reactions [see ✏ p. 162 box].

β_2-antagonists. There are no really selective β_2-antagonists, and in general, one does not want to block the β_2-receptors on smooth muscle; the exception is preparation of a patient with phaeochromocytoma for surgery, when propranalol (with the β-blocker phenoxybenzamine) may be used to protect the patient from the effects of a surge of catecholamines during removal of the tumour [see ✏ p. 164]. β-blockers are important antihypertensive, anti-anginal and antidysrhythmic agents [see ✏ Tables 7.4, 14.5, 13.1, 13.2]; in most of these, the β_1-blocking action is the fundamental effect.

α_1- and β-antagonist, labetalol (not shown): for hypertension, phaeochromocytoma [see ✏ Table 7.4].

Agents acting on the noradrenergic neuron:

Guanethidine, a noradrenergic neuron blocker: for hypertension [see ✏ Tables 7.4, 14.4].

Methyldopa, gives rise to false transmitter methylnoradrenaline: an α_2-agonist used in hypertension [see ✏ p. 175 box].

Carbidopa, inhibitor of dopa decarboxylase: adjunct to L-dopa therapy

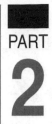

PART

2

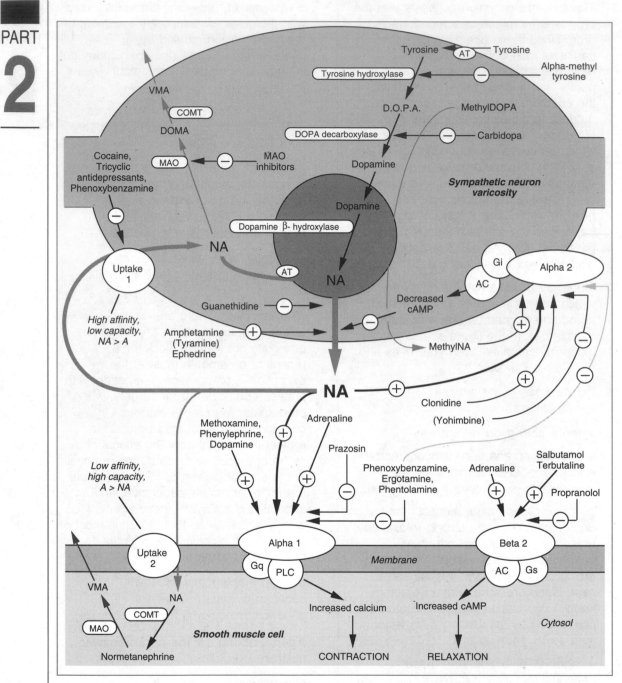

Fig. 32 The main transduction events at the junction of sympathetic neuron and smooth muscle, giving the main drugs which affect synthesis, release, re-uptake and action of noradrenaline (NA). A = adrenaline; G = G-protein (Gs: stimulatory, Gi: inhibitory); AC = adenylate cyclase; PLC = phospholipase C; AT = active transport. In some smooth muscle, activation of the alpha 2 receptor opens an ion channel and the influx of sodium causes membrane depolarisation which activates voltage-dependent calcium channels [see Fig. 21 in this book]. The pathways of metabolism of NA have been simplified; for more detail see Fig. 8.5.

of parkinsonism, prevents peripheral sympathomimetic effects which could occur if L-dopa were converted to dopamine and then to NA [see 📖 pp. 529, 167].

Methyltyrosine, inhibitor of tyrosine hydroxylase: occasionally used in phaeochromocytoma [see 📖 Table 7.4, p. 167].

Ephedrine, displaces NA from neuron: nasal decongestant [see 📖 p. 162 box].

Amphetamine, displaces NA from neuron: used for narcolepsy [see 📖 p. 639, Table 7.4].

33. **A.** True; aspirin has an antiplatelet effect and may also displace warfarin from plasma proteins [see 📖 p. 338, Table 4.1]. The interaction could lead to bleeding.

B. False; it increases the effect. Amphetamine is sympathomimetic, by virtue of displacing NA from noradrenergic neurons. The NA is then taken up back into the neuron where some is metabolised by monoamine oxidase (MAO), type A. Tranylcypromine is a MAO inhibitor and will increase NA content in neurons and thus its subsequent actions. A hypertensive crisis could result from this interaction. (Note that amphetamines are not used extensively in clinical treatment but they may be used in the drug culture) [see 📖 p. 590].

C. True; aspirin interferes with the plasma protein binding of tolbutamide [see 📖 Table 4.1] and may also decrease its metabolism by competing with metabolising enzymes. Since tolbutamide works at a plasma concentration at which the binding to protein is approaching saturation, the above actions of aspirin will increase the concentration of free tolbutamide and thus increase its hypoglycaemic effect [see 📖 p. 415].

D. False; LTD_4 is a spasmogen causing contraction by the mechanisms detailed

in Chapter 41. It is a mediator of bronchospasm in asthma. Terbutaline is a β_2-agonist on smooth muscle causing relaxation by the mechanisms detailed in Chapter 41. Terbutaline will reduce the effect of LTD by acting as a physiological antagonist; it is used as a bronchodilator in the therapy of asthma [see 📖 Fig. 17.3, pp. 359, 17].

E. True; the combination of these two antidepressant agents can result in high fever, high blood pressure and marked CNS excitation. The exact mechanism is not known [see 📖 p. 590].

34. Prednisone is an anti-inflammatory and immunosuppressive glucocorticoid which is inactive until converted by metabolism to prednisolone [see 📖 Table 21.2].

Lithium is used to control mania. Its action is not increased by metabolism; it is excreted virtually unchanged in the urine [see 📖 p. 594].

Azathioprine, used as an immunosuppressant, is a pro-drug which is inactive until metabolised to mercaptopurine [see 📖 p. 263].

Methicillin is a β-lactamase-resistant penicillin active against Gram-positive cocci (but not against Gram-negative bacteria). It is not rendered more active by metabolism; 88% is excreted unchanged in the urine.

Cyclophosphamide is an immunosuppressant and anticancer drug which is metabolised in the liver to aldophosphamide which is subsequently converted in the tissue to phosphoramide mustard—the actual cytotoxic moiety [see 📖 Fig. 36.6].

Glyceryl trinitrate is an anti-anginal drug. If swallowed it would be virtually completely inactivated by metabolism in the liver. It has to be given sublingually [see 📖 p. 295]. However, when so given it releases nitrite ion which is converted to nitric oxide which is the active agent—it causes vasodilatation by activating

PART

2

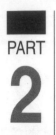

guanylate cyclase [see Ch. 41, and 📖 Fig. 13.15].

Paracetamol has antipyretic and analgesic properties, being used for headache and other pains associated with vascular changes [see 📖 p. 255 box]. It does not require metabolism in order to produce its effects. If taken in excessive doses, which saturate the

normal conjugation reactions, it is metabolised to an active compound, N-acetyl-p-benzoquinone imine, but since this is seriously toxic it cannot be regarded as a clinically desirable effect [see 📖 Figs 12.1B, 43.1].

35. a. Figure 33 shows the main receptors and some of the initial transduction events which occur at the junction of

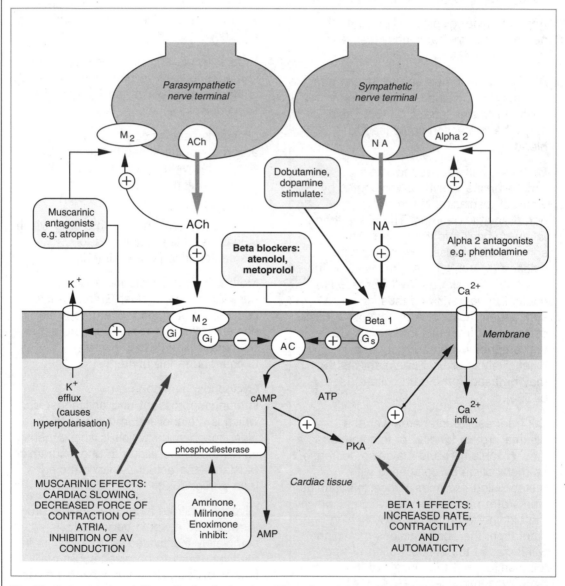

Fig. 33 Autonomic transmitter action on the heart and the action of drugs. Muscarinic M_2 effects occur mostly in the atrium and nodal tissue. Beta 1 effects occur in the pacemaker, nodal tissue and muscle. Dobutamine has more inotropic than chronotropic action. AC = adenylate cyclase; G = G-protein (Gs: stimulatory, Gi: inhibitory); PKA = cAMP-activated protein kinase.

postganglionic autonomic nerves and cardiac tissue and indicates some relevant drug actions. Drugs with important clinical uses are shown in bold type.

β-blockers are used in angina, hypertension, cardiac dysrhythmias and myocardial infarction [see 📖 p. 166 box].

Phosphodiesterase inhibitors (e.g. milrinone) can be used, short term, for congestive heart failure which has not responded to more conventional drugs [see 📖 p. 286].

Dopamine and dobutamine have more inotropic than chronotropic effect and are infused i.v. in cardiogenic shock [see 📖 Table 14.3, Fig. 14.10]. Note that dopamine also acts on dopamine receptors in renal and mesenteric arteries and receptors in other blood vessels [see 📖 p. 309].

Muscarinic antagonists have many actions [see 📖 p. 128]. In the context of the heart, atropine is used as part of the therapy of profound bradycardia, also to overcome excessive action of an anticholinesterase and, occasionally, in patients in whom excessive vagal tone is compromising therapy of cardiac dysfunction.

b. The non-selective α-blockers, phenoxybenzamine and phentolamine, are the agents whose inhibitory action on α_1-receptors in blood vessels might be thought to be of value in hypertension. However, if these antagonists on both α_2- and α_1-receptors were to be used to treat hypertension, their α_1-blocking effect in the blood vessels might lead to decreased vasoconstriction by noradrenaline and might tend to reduce blood pressure, were it not for the effect shown here, namely the action on the α_2-receptors. Stimulation of these receptors prevents the normal negative feedback effect of noradrenaline and thus results in increased noradrenaline release and, therefore, increased rate and force of

contraction of the heart as a result of the action of noradrenaline on cardiac β_1-receptors; this counteracts the vasodilator effects. Phenoxybenzamine, given orally, can be used short term, with a β-blocker for episodes of phaeochromocytoma-induced hypertension [see 📖 p. 164].

36. The main transduction events are shown schematically in Figure 34, as are the main drugs which could influence the events.

The benzodiazepines are used as anxiolytics and hypnotics and as anti-epileptic agents. Diazepam is also used for basal anaesthesia [see 📖 pp. 605, 543].

Flumazenil, a benzodiazepine antagonist, is employed to overcome the effects of benzodiazepine overdose and may have a role in reversing the sedative action of benzodiazepines used during anaesthesia [see 📖 p. 558].

Barbiturates: thiopentone is an intravenous anaesthetic, phenobarbitone is used as an antiepileptic [see 📖 p. 544, Table 30.1].

Phenytoin, valproate and vigabatrin are antiepileptics [see 📖 Table 30.1].

Baclofen is a centrally acting muscle relaxant [see 📖 pp. 607–608].

Phaclofen, muscimol, bicuculline, picrotoxin and the inverse agonists are experimental tools [see 📖 pp. 514 box, 555].

37. The main eicosanoid of importance in normal endothelium/platelet interaction is prostacyclin (PGI_2) [see Fig. 35(1)]. An outline of the role of eicosanoids in the specific interaction between platelets and atherosclerotic plaque is given in Figure 35(2a). The likely result of such an interaction in the coronary arterial system is arterial thrombosis with resultant myocardial infarction. Drugs which could modify the processes outlined are given

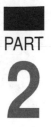

PART

2

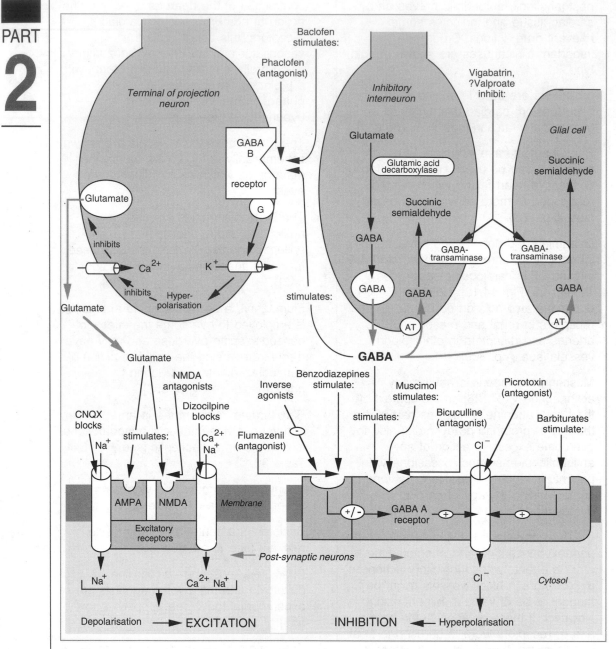

Fig. 34 Summary diagram of drugs acting on the GABA and glutamate systems. A schematic diagram of part of a glial cell, a neuronal terminal releasing glutamate and an interneuron releasing GABA, showing GABA synthesis and re-uptake, the receptors for GABA and glutamate with the main transduction events following receptor activation, and the drugs which affect these processes. Inverse agonists have both stimulant and antagonist actions. AT = active transport; G = G-protein; NMDA = N-methyl-D-aspartate.

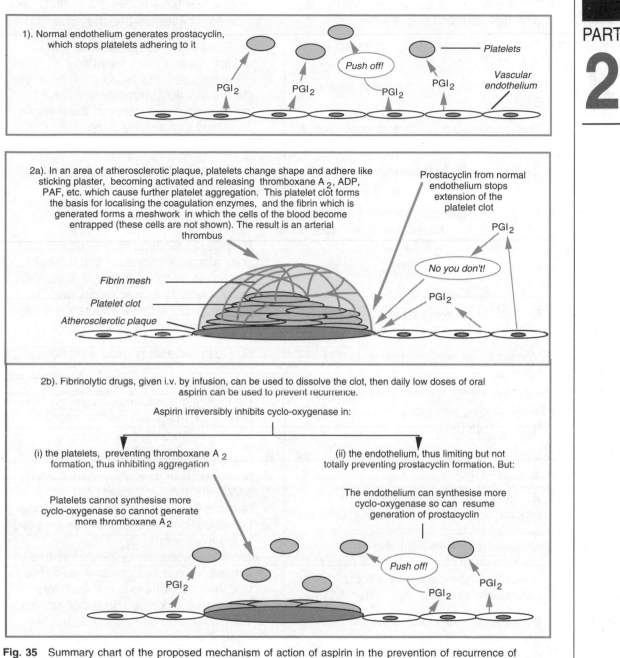

Fig. 35 Summary chart of the proposed mechanism of action of aspirin in the prevention of recurrence of myocardinal infarction. PGI$_2$ = prostacyclin.

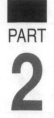

in Figures 11 and 35(2b) [see also pp. 342, 344, 348 box, Fig. 16.10].

38. Pralidoxime and atropine for dyflos [see p. 144].

Protamine sulphate for heparin [see p. 341].

Tranexamic acid for streptokinase [see p. 348].

Carbidopa with levodopa [see p. 529 box].

Mesna for cyclophosphamide (it interacts with the toxic metabolite, acrolein) [see p. 706 box].

Naloxone for morphine [see p. 631 box].

Methionine for paracetamol [see p. 255].

Vitamin K_1 for warfarin [see p. 335 box].

Neostigmine for tubocurarine (*not for suxamethonium*) [see Table 6.7, Fig. 6.8B, p. 145 box].

Desferrioxamine for ferrous sulphate [see p. 478 box].

39. A. True; with many penicillins, the amount excreted via the urine is 80% or more (remember the story of the first clinical use of penicillin) and renal impairment might increase the risk of unwanted hypersensitivity effects, rashes particularly [see p. 727, Table 4.6].

B. False; atenolol is excreted virtually unchanged in the urine and would cumulate if kidney function were impaired. The dose must be adjusted [see Table 4.6]. Note that renal function would, by definition, be impaired in the hypertension which is secondary to renal disease, and atenolol might well be a first-line drug for treatment of this condition.

C. True; labetalol is metabolised in the liver; it undergoes substantial first-pass

metabolism [see Tables 4.3, 7.4]. Less than 5% is eliminated in the urine.

D. False; it would be necessary to reduce dosage since for many cephalosporins the amount excreted via the urine is 80% or more, and renal impairment would increase the risk of unwanted effects [see pp. 728–729, Table 4.6].

E. False; cromoglycate is given by inhalation and only about 10% is absorbed into the circulation [see p. 363 box].

F. True; elimination of aminoglycosides is by glomerular filtration and if renal function is impaired they will cumulate; this will lead to nephrotoxicity and ototoxicity since these effects are dose-related [see p. 733].

G. False; ethanol is more than 90% metabolised, the remainder being excreted in the breath and the urine. Renal impairment would therefore have only a minimal effect on the plasma concentration [see p. 658].

40. General inhibitors of the phosphodiesterase which metabolises cAMP are the xanthine drugs (theophylline, enprofylline). These have bronchodilator actions and may be used in the treatment of the bronchoconstriction of the first phase of asthma. (There is also some evidence that they might have some inhibitory action on the delayed phase of asthma.) They have mild diuretic action but are rarely if ever used as diuretics now [see p. 360 box].

Amrinone, milrinone and enoximone have specific inotropic actions which are believed to be due to their acting more selectively on iso-enzymes of the cAMP phosphodiesterase which occur in the heart [see Fig. 33]. They are used in cardiac failure (but recent evidence suggests that they might increase mortality) [see p. 286].

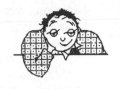

PART

2

41. A. True [see 📖 p. 502 box].

B. False; it causes increased tone of GIT muscle and decreases peristalsis. It can be used to treat diarrhoea [see 📖 p. 399].

C. False; these two new antihistamine drugs (and also mequitazine) do not have sedative effects; previously developed H_1-antagonists (diphenhydramine, promethazine) are sedative [see 📖 Table 12.4].

D. False.
Don't even
think of trying it
[see 📖 p. 638, footnote].

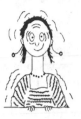

E. True [see 📖 p. 514 box].

F. False; the barbiturates used for I.v. anaesthesia are thiopentone and methohexitone [see 📖 p. 546 box]. Phenobarbitone is used as an anticonvulsant [see 📖 p. 560].

G. False; it is used for all types of epilepsy except absence seizures [see 📖 Table 30.1].

H. True [see 📖 Fig. 19.8].

I. False on several counts. Current evidence is that dextropropoxyphene is not even as potent as codeine and it has addiction liability [see 📖 p. 629]. Overdosage with the combination will produce both serious paracetamol-induced liver damage [see 📖 Fig. 43.1] and also dextropropoxyphene-induced respiratory depression.

J. True [see 📖 pp. 568–569, Fig. 28.3].

K. (i) False; it is metabolised by zero-order kinetics [see 📖 Figs 4.24, 33.5].

(ii) False; it is distributed throughout the body water.

(iii) True [see 📖 p. 655].

(iv) –

(v) False.
Worrablurryshame!
[see 📖 p. 655].

42. Antagonism of fast excitatory transmission such as that which occurs at the AMPA (non-NMDA) receptors for glutamate and aspartate would cause a massive depression of the CNS. The reason is that most cells in the brain use glutamate as a neuro-transmitter and fast transmission at AMPA receptors is critical for point-to-point communication between neurons. CNQX is an antagonist at this receptor. Conversely, inhibiting fast GABA inhibition which is mediated by the $GABA_A$ receptor would produce overstimulation of the CNS and convulsions. Bicuculline is an antagonist at this receptor [see 📖 pp. 511, 512 box, 514 box, Table 24.3].

43. Yes, by using NMDA receptors for glutamate as a target and the ability of benzodiazepines to enhance $GABA_A$-mediated inhibition. The complex voltage- and ligand-gated NMDA receptor is not involved in fast transmission under normal situations. Drugs based on agents such as AP5 (receptor antagonist) and ketamine and MK801 (channel blockers) could be useful antiepileptic, antineurodegenerative and sedative agents. They may also be useful for pain relief. The benzodiazepines, by actions on their own site, enhance GABA transmission and are used as antiepileptics, anxiolytics, sedatives and muscle relaxants [see 📖 pp. 512 box, 514 box].

44. The circumstances would be a surgical operation. Diazepam would be given preoperatively to reduce anxiety and cause a degree of muscle relaxation. Morphine would be given to reduce anxiety and as an analgesic both before and after the operation depending on the case. Atropine would be given preoperatively to inhibit the bronchial

PART

2

secretions induced by inhalation anaesthetics. Thiopentone would be injected intravenously to induce anaesthesia but, because of its short half-life and redistribution to fat, halothane would then be given continuously by inhalation to maintain anaesthesia. Tubocurarine would be given to produce muscle relaxation since it is a competitive nicotinic antagonist at the neuromuscular junction.

45. Depression is thought to result from *reduced* noradrenaline levels leading to receptor upregulation. Parkinson's disease results from a *loss* of dopamine neurons in the striatum.

In each of these two cases, there is a deficit which treatment aims to restore, by decreasing either uptake or breakdown of noradrenaline by tricyclic drugs or MAOIs respectively, in the case of depression, or by increased availability of dopamine (with levodopa) in the case of Parkinson's disease.

Anxiety, schizophrenia, pain and epilepsy can all be considered as being due to *too much activity* in the neural systems, and treatment is aimed at reducing this. Thus in the case of anxiety, GABA inhibition is increased by the use of benzodiazepines. This approach is also effective in epilepsy. Increasing inhibitory transmission by opioid agonists is used in pain as is the decreasing excitation by blocking of prostaglandin synthesis by NSAIDs and the blocking of peripheral neuronal excitation with local anaesthetics. Blocking excitation with phenytoin or increasing GABA inhibition with barbiturates are also effective tactics in treating epilepsy. Finally, antagonists at dopamine receptors are helpful in the treatment of schizophrenia. Thus the excess activity can be reduced either by antagonising excitation, or by increasing inhibition.

Appendix

LIST OF THE MAIN PHARMACOLOGICAL AGENTS

Many students feel overwhelmed by the inordinate number of drugs dealt with in pharmacology textbooks. To lighten the burden we list on pages 179–182 the more important pharmacological agents. The list is divided into agents of primary importance and those of secondary importance. In general, pharmacology courses require a detailed knowledge of the drugs in the first category, including actions and mode of action, and (for those used therapeutically) pharmacokinetic properties, side effects, toxicity and main uses. For drugs in the second category, a knowledge of the mechanism of action is usually sufficient, and also, where appropriate, an understanding of how they differ from those in the primary category. We have included not only drugs used therapeutically but also endogenous chemical mediators/transmitters and certain important drugs used as experimental tools.

But note that this list is only a general guide to necessary drugs. Different pharmacology departments may leave out some of our examples while stressing others, depending on the relative emphasis on 'clinical usage' as compared to 'mechanism of action' of drugs in their courses. For example, there was inevitably some divergence in the lists of drugs suggested by pharmacologists and by clinicians who were asked to vet this section.

Primary	Secondary

PERIPHERAL NERVOUS SYSTEM (PNS)
Drugs acting on ACh receptors

Primary	Secondary
acetylcholine	carbachol pilocarpine
atropine	hyoscine (scopolamine) pirenzepine homatropine ipratropium cyclopentolate
tubocurarine	trimetaphan
suxamethonium (succinylcholine)	pancuronium atracurium

Anticholinesterases

Primary	Secondary
neostigmine	edrophonium eserine (physostigmine) DFP pralidoxime (antidote)

Drugs acting on the noradrenergic neuron and adrenoceptors

Primary	Secondary
adrenaline	clonidine
noradrenaline	phenylephrine
isoprenaline	tyramine amphetamine (see CNS)
salbutamol	terbutaline
atenolol	
propranolol	
dobutamine	
	phentolamine yohimbine
prazosin	phenoxybenzamine labetalol
guanethidine	α-methyl tyrosine methyldopa cocaine imipramine (see CNS) phenelzine (see CNS)

Local anaesthetics (LAs)

Primary	Secondary
lignocaine	bupivacaine

CARDIOVASCULAR SYSTEM
Antidysrhythmic drugs

Primary	Secondary
digoxin	
lignocaine (see also LAs)	
propranolol (see also PNS)	sotalol quinidine
verapamil	disopyramide
amiodarone	

Anti-anginal drugs

Primary	Secondary
propranolol (see PNS)	
nifedipine	amlodipine diltiazem
glyceryl trinitrate	isosorbide dinitrate

Antihypertensive drugs

Primary	Secondary
atenolol	
propranolol (see also PNS)	hydralazine
diuretics (see also kidney)	
	doxazosin
captopril	enalapril minoxidil
nifedipine	nitroprusside methyldopa (see also PNS) clonidine (see also PNS) labetalol (see also PNS)

Drugs used in acute heart failure

Primary	Secondary
dobutamine	dopamine
frusemide	
morphine	

Drugs used in chronic heart failure

Primary	Secondary
thiazides, frusemide (see also kidney)	
digoxin	
nitrates	
captopril	enalapril

PERIPHERAL CIRCULATION
(see also under noradrenergic neuron, anti-anginal drugs, antihypertensives)

Primary	Secondary
angiotensin	
dopamine	
	ergotamine endothelin nitric oxide (endothelium-derived-relaxing factor, EDRF)

KIDNEY

Primary	Secondary
bendrofluazide	mannitol
frusemide	aldosterone spironolactone amiloride
vasopressin (ADH)	desmopressin probenecid potassium citrate ammonium chloride

PART 2

Primary	Secondary

CENTRAL NERVOUS SYSTEM
Neurotransmitters

Primary	Secondary
glutamate	
dopamine	acetylcholine
GABA	noradrenaline
glycine	various peptides
5-HT	

General anaesthetics
Inhalation

Primary	Secondary
nitrous oxide	
halothane	
enflurane	isoflurane

Intravenous

Primary	Secondary
thiopentone	propofol ketamine etomidate

Hypnotics and anxiolytics

Primary	Secondary
temazepam	diazepam
nitrazepam	buspirone

Analgesics and narcotic antagonists

Primary	Secondary
morphine	codeine fentanyl methadone diamorphine (heroin) pethidine
enkephalins	β-endorphin dynorphin
naloxone	
aspirin paracetamol }	(see under Local hormones)

Antidepressants and antimanic drugs

Primary	Secondary
amitriptyline	fluoxetine
imipramine	mianserin
phenelzine	moclobemide
lithium	

Neuroleptics

Primary	Secondary
chlorpromazine	haloperidol
clozapine	flupenthixol
thioridazine	sulpiride

Drugs which may cause dependence/abuse

Primary	Secondary
barbiturates	lysergic acid diethylamide (LSD)
heroin	
cocaine	
alcohol	nicotine
cannabis	
amphetamine	
L-methylinedioxyamphetamine (ecstasy)	
	anabolic steroids

Anti-emetics

Primary	Secondary
hyoscine	cyclizine
metoclopramide	prochlorperazine
ondansetron	

Drugs affecting motor disorders, parkinsonism, epilepsy, etc

Primary	Secondary
phenytoin	phenobarbitone
carbamazepine	
sodium valproate	diazepam
clonazepam	ethosuximide
levodopa	benzhexol
carbidopa	selegiline bromocriptine

THE ENDOCRINE SYSTEM
Drugs affecting the pancreas and carbohydrate metabolism

Primary	Secondary
Insulin preparations: • soluble • isophane • protamine zinc	glucagon
metformin	
tolbutamide	glibenclamide

Thyroid hormones and antithyroid drugs

Primary	Secondary
thyroxine	liothyronine
iodide	propylthiouracil
carbimazole	
	radioiodine ^{131}I

Lipid-lowering drugs

Primary	Secondary
simvastatin	cholestyramine bezafibrate gemfibrosil

Primary	Secondary
Anterior pituitary/adrenal	
prednisolone	beclomethasone (for asthma, skin conditions)
hydrocortisone	
fludrocortisone	
corticotrophin (ACTH)	
Anterior pituitary	
growth hormone	
	octreotide
Hypothalamus/sex hormones	
ethinyloestradiol	norethisterone
progesterone	
testosterone	
	tamoxifen
	busrelin
	urofollitrophin
Uterus	
ergometrine	
oxytocin	
	ritodrine
dinoprostone	
	NSAIDs (see also Local hormones)
BLOOD COAGULATION AND THROMBOSIS	
aspirin	dipyridamole
heparin	protamine sulphate
warfarin	
phytomenadione (vit. K$_1$)	
	prostacyclin
	thromboxane A$_2$
streptokinase	anistreplase
HAEMOPOIESIS	
Ferrous sulphate	
Folic acid	
Vitamin B$_{12}$	
Erythropoietin	
Monocyte/granulocyte colony-stimulating factors	

Primary	Secondary
LOCAL HORMONES AND THEIR ANTAGONISTS, NSAIDS AND OTHER DRUGS USED TO TREAT INFLAMMATION	
histamine	
chlorpheniramine	
astemizole	terfenadine
5-hydroxytryptamine	methysergide
	pizotifen
bradykinin	
	cromoglycate
prostaglandins thromboxanes prostacyclin leukotrienes } eicosanoids	
aspirin	indomethacin
paracetamol	ibuprofen
	penicillamine
	auranofin
allopurinol	probenecid
glucocorticoids (see under Anterior pituitary/adrenal)	
GASTROINTESTINAL TRACT	
ranitidine	cimetidine
	omeprazole
	misoprostol
	sucralfate
magnesium trisilicate	pirenzepine
	aluminium hydroxide
senna	loperamide
methylcellulose	magnesium sulphate

To eliminate *Helicobacter pylori*:
bismuth plus omeprazole plus clarithromycin

CANCER CHEMOTHERAPY	
cyclophosphamide	cytarabine
methotrexate	mercaptopurine
doxorubicin	fluorouracil
	vincristine
	cisplatin
	etoposide

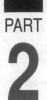

PART

2

Primary	Secondary

IMMUNOSUPPRESSANTS

Primary	Secondary
cyclosporin	cyclophosphamide (see also Cancer)
azathioprine	methotrexate (see also Cancer)
	antilymphocyte globulin
prednisolone (see also Adrenal)	

RESPIRATORY TRACT

salbutamol (see also PNS)	
salmeterol	
aminophylline	cromoglycate (see also Local hormones)
beclomethasone	
budesonide	
ipratropium bromide	
	codeine (see also Analgesics)

CHEMOTHERAPY

Antibacterial agents

benzylpenicillin	cephalosporins
flucloxacillin	ciprofloxacin
amoxycillin	sulphonamides
azlocillin	chloramphenicol
erythromycin	
gentamicin	
tetracycline	
trimethoprim	

Antimycobacterial agents

isoniazid	dapsone
rifampicin	ethambutol
pyrazinamide	streptomycin

Antiviral agents

acyclovir	tribavirin
zidovudine	ganciclovir

Primary	Secondary

Antiprotozoal agents

For malaria:

chloroquine	pyrimethamine plus sulphadoxine
quinine	

For Pneumocystis carinii:

co-trimoxazole (high dose)

pentamidine

For amoebiasis:

metronidazole

diloxanide furoate

For leishmaniasis :

sodium stibogluconate

For trypanosomiasis:

pentamidine

Anthelminthics

mebendazole

niclosamide

pyrantel

diethylcarbamazine

Antifungal agents

fluconazole	nystatin
amphotericin	griseofulvin flucytosine